SWING FLAWS
AND
FITNESS FIXES

SWING FLAWS
AND
FITNESS FIXES

Fix Your Swing by Putting Flexibility, Strength, and Stamina in Your Golf Bag

KATHERINE ROBERTS

GOTHAM
BOOKS

Every effort has been made to ensure that the information contained in this book is complete and accurate. However, neither the author nor the publisher is engaged in rendering professional advice or services to the individual reader. The ideas, procedures, and suggestions contained in this book are not intended as a substitute for consulting with your physician. All matters regarding your health require medical supervision. Neither the author nor the publisher shall be liable or responsible for any loss, injury, or damage allegedly arising from any information or suggestions in this book.

GOTHAM BOOKS
Published by Penguin Group (USA) Inc.
375 Hudson Street, New York, New York 10014, U.S.A.

Penguin Group (Canada), 90 Eglinton Avenue East, Suite 700, Toronto, Ontario M4P 2Y3, Canada (a division of Pearson Penguin Canada Inc.); Penguin Books Ltd, 80 Strand, London WC2R 0RL, England; Penguin Ireland, 25 St Stephen's Green, Dublin 2, Ireland (a division of Penguin Books Ltd); Penguin Group (Australia), 250 Camberwell Road, Camberwell, Victoria 3124, Australia (a division of Pearson Australia Group Pty Ltd); Penguin Books India Pvt Ltd, 11 Community Centre, Panchsheel Park, New Delhi—110 017, India; Penguin Group (NZ), 67 Apollo Drive, Rosedale, North Shore 0632, New Zealand (a division of Pearson New Zealand Ltd); Penguin Books (South Africa) (Pty) Ltd, 24 Sturdee Avenue, Rosebank, Johannesburg 2196, South Africa

Penguin Books Ltd, Registered Offices: 80 Strand, London WC2R 0RL, England

Published by Gotham Books, a member of Penguin Group (USA) Inc.

First printing, August 2009
10   9   8   7   6   5   4   3   2   1

Photos by Jaime Kowal Photography, Vancouver, British Columbia. All images were selected by Matt Carothers of The Green Room (www.greenroomgolf.com) and were provided by Jon Nason of Motion Reality, Inc. (www.motionrealityinc.com).

Gotham Books and the skyscraper logo are trademarks of Penguin Group (USA) Inc.

LIBRARY OF CONGRESS CATALOGING-IN-PUBLICATION DATA
Roberts, Katherine (Katherine J.), 1962–
    Swing flaws and fitness fixes: fix your swing by putting flexibility, strength, and stamina in your golf bag / Katherine Roberts.
        p.   cm.
    ISBN 978-1-592-40456-8 (pbk.)
1. Swing (Golf)   2. Golf—Training.   3. Physical fitness.   I. Title.
    GV979.S9R6 2009
    796.352'3—dc22   2009009030

Printed in the United States of America
Set in Adobe Caslon, with News Gothic and Felix Tilting
Designed by BTDNYC

While the author has made every effort to provide accurate telephone numbers and Internet addresses at the time of publication, neither the publisher nor the author assumes any responsibility for errors, or for changes that occur after publication. Further, the publisher does not have any control over and does not assume any responsibility for author or third-party Web sites or their content.

FOR MY HUSBAND, MARK

YOUR INTELLIGENCE, HUMOR,
ENCOURAGEMENT, AND
UNCONDITIONAL LOVE
ARE A DAILY BLESSING

CONTENTS

Chapter Twelve: Casting/Scooping the Ball

Casting occurs as a breakdown in the swing during the downswing. Typically it is caused when the angle of the wrists is released too early. The proper fix for casting is to evaluate the mobility, stability, and strength of the lower body, the action from the shoulders and wrists, and the kinematic sequence.

> 3D analysis
>
> Hank's perspective
>
> Fitness solutions

Chapter Thirteen: Chicken Wing

The chicken wing occurs when the left arm bends at impact and continues bending to the finish position. The result is a decrease of power, distance, and accuracy. Physical restrictions causing this flaw are the issues of shoulder and trunk inflexibility, a lack of shoulder turn, and an inability to properly initiate the lower body in the downswing.

> 3D analysis
>
> Hank's perspective
>
> Fitness solutions

Chapter Fourteen: Reverse "C" Spine Angle

The "reverse C" is defined as a finish position in which the upper body is bent backward and laterally toward the target. Golfers with a "reverse C" flaw have a tendency to hook the ball and at the same time put tremendous stress on the lower back. For most golfers this position is a manifestation of weak core stabilization.

> 3D analysis
>
> Hank's perspective
>
> Fitness solutions

SECTION THREE—THE ROBERTS FLEX-FIT METHOD FOR A STRONGER BODY AND LOWER SCORES

Chapter Fifteen: Build Your Back Strength

Poor swing mechanics places a repetitive strain on the body and tremendous pressure on the lumbar spine, causing back pain. Since some 53 percent of golfers play with low back pain and as many as 30 percent of touring pros play injured, focusing our attention on building a healthy back is critical for peak performance. Off the course, back pain contributes to more lost work days and analgesic consumption than any other physical complaint. In addition to targeting the lower back, this series targets spine flexibility and hip and hamstring mobility—all of which contribute to a healthy back—and offers a number of strengthening exercises.

Chapter Sixteen: Core Stability and Strength— The Fundamental of Golf Fitness

Developing a strong core facilitates more consistency and better posture. This chapter focuses on creating a stable, strong core by incorporating exercises for the deepest part of the abdominals, the muscles of the entire back, and the glutes.

Chapter Seventeen: Balance, Proprioception, Vision, and Foot Function

A balanced golf swing is a goal of every golfer. A solid golf shot begins with balance at address and continues through the swing and into the finish position. In this chapter we examine movement, proprioception, understanding the impact of vision, and the role of foot function in your swing. Proper foot function is important for walking the course without fatigue, maintaining balance, and ensuring the efficient transference of ground forces from the lower body to the club.

Two important and rarely emphasized components of golf performance is the concept of recovery and rest. Scientific research proves the benefits of post-round and pre-rest stretching. Restorative exercises support the renewal of broken-down muscle fibers, while passive stretching reduces soreness. This series of exercises benefits you physically as well as mentally. Refueling offers you tips and guidelines for nutrition and hydration.

ACKNOWLEDGMENTS & CONTRIBUTIONS

First and foremost I want to thank Hank Haney, the consummate teacher, for his insights on the golf swing and for the many hours we spent together on the practice tee discussing golf and life. Secondly I want to thank Hank, my friend, for coaching me on the significance of following my passion.

Dr. Alan Reichow, Nike's Global Research Director for Vision Science, has graciously shared his vast knowledge of the importance of vision and golf performance. You opened my eyes (pun intended) to "sensory fitness."

There are many other people who deserve to be acknowledged for their efforts in the evolution of this book. Thank you to Matt Carothers, CPGA professional from The Green Room Golf Performance Center, Vancouver, British Columbia, for providing the 3D motion-capture images (MotionRealityInc.com) and for his input as one of our fitness models. Jim Budd, another one of our fitness models who at the age of fifty-five is the Senior Club Champion for The Sunshine Coast Golf Club in Roberts Creek, British Columbia. Jim is my role model for limitless possibilities, on and off the course.

Thank you to William Shinker, my publisher, and Patrick Mulligan, my editor from Gotham. Thanks to my agent, John Monteleone. Your humor always brings me back to my senses.

I want to thank Deb Mealia for her grounding insights, and my mother, Ruth Gordon, for always believing I can achieve anything (as long as I don't think or act like a sheep).

Lastly, I want to send love to my dogs Max, Simba, and Cayla. Thank you for encouraging me to take long walks in the woods and for reminding me not to take myself too seriously.

FOREWORD

OLF IS OFTEN considered to be the most difficult game in the world. Having taught more than fifty thousand golf lessons over the last thirty-two years, I would have to agree. Why is golf so tough? I think there are many reasons. For one thing, the ball is small and the clubhead isn't very big—the margin of error in hitting a golf ball isn't much, and if your clubface is off just a degree or two the ball isn't going to go where you want it to go. Another factor that makes golf so hard is that the mechanics of the golf swing are very complicated, difficult to understand, hard to teach, and even harder to learn. But the one thing I see every day as a teacher that makes golf so hard is that a lot of people can't physically do what they are trying to do in the golf swing. This is why when I was doing my ESPN Golf Schools I always had Katherine Roberts doing her fitness for golf as part of my program. I always felt that if Katherine had a chance to work with my students, she would in turn give me a chance to accomplish what I was trying to do with the mechanical changes that I thought my students needed to make in their swings. As a teacher, I've found that it's one thing to know what a student needs to do to improve; getting them to do it is another story. There are always hurdles that any student or teacher has to overcome, but physically not being able to do something is the biggest roadblock that anyone trying to learn and execute an effective golf swing can come up against.

There are four areas of physical conditioning that will play a part in any golfer's ability to play the game well. The first is properly warming up before every practice session or round of golf. The second is building your strength, speed, and stability so that you can apply those attributes to your swing. The third area is being able to make a full swing and being able to coil properly. And the fourth is having the physical stamina to stay physically and mentally in shape for at least eighteen holes of golf.

Golf is a physical activity, and if you want to play your best you really need to be in good physical shape. There are two factors involved in playing the game of golf: distance and direction. Distance is the factor that to the greatest extent determines a player's potential. This is evidenced by the fact that even on the PGA Tour, where all the players are obviously highly skilled, the longest hitters are the ones who dominate the game. This hasn't gone unnoticed, and thus working out and improving one's strength is a big part of virtually every player's training program. Better strength and faster muscles will mean more speed to any golfer, and more speed means more distance. One of the most important conditioning activities that players and trainers always work on is strengthening the player's core muscles. You will find that Katherine Roberts' program will focus on building a more stable core. When you have a more stable and stronger core, everything that you try to do in the golf swing will be easier to do.

Probably the most inhibiting factor in any golfer's ability to make a good golf swing is a lack of flexibility. Some people are just prone to be tight physically, while others tend to get tight when they work out. And regardless of body type, everyone loses flexibility with age. I have seen just about every different kind of golf swing over the years, and the one thing that I see over and over again is players who are too tight and who simply can't make a full or proper pivot in the golf swing. When you aren't able to move properly, it goes without saying that you can't swing powerfully or properly. Katherine Roberts' Flex-Fit Method is an easy and patient approach to improving any golfer's flexibility. Her program combines simple stretches with core stabilization and strengthening, and they all employ her special breathing techniques that really make everything work.

The last factor that I think every golfer should consider is that the better overall condition you are in, the more you'll be able to maintain your level of play throughout an entire round. Additionally, I have always believed that one round of tournament golf is more physically taxing than thirty-six holes of recreational golf, due to the amount of mental energy that you put into a round of competition. It is for this reason that the better shape you're in, the stronger you'll be throughout a round of golf—not to mention a whole tournament. The more physically fit you are, the more mentally fit you will be.

I really believe that this book by Katherine Roberts will give you the help you need to take your golf game to a new level. There is no chance that if you work on some of the simple exercises that Katherine recommends that you won't improve your game. I have seen Katherine and her programs help so many golfers that I know she will do the same for you. I know this because she has even helped me.

—Hank Haney

INTRODUCTION

SINCE MAN'S FIRST round, the quest for the perfect swing has consumed golfers. Have you taken lessons, spent countless dollars on the newest equipment, practiced for hours with little or no improvement? Have you tried to contort your body into the "proper" position but found that your body simply will not cooperate?

Imagine yourself in the finish position—what one Top 100 teacher called the "world-class finish" position—with your belly button facing the target and your eyes tracking the flight of the ball. Are you upright and in balance? Are you turned and facing the target with eyes and head level? Or are you teetering and toppling like a toddler taking his first steps?

A swing flaw is a physiological breakdown in one or more of the various phases of the golf swing. These breakdowns contribute to a loss of power and distance, contribute to inconsistency, and often cause physical injury. When you are not operating at your optimal levels of mobility, stability, and strength and not physically capable of executing an efficient swing, flaws occur.

Knowledge facilitates power and awareness. Awareness creates change.

In Chapter One you will learn about the specific muscles activated during various phases of the golf swing and the importance of an efficient kinetic link. The kinetic link defines the transference of energy in the body that is responsible for power in the swing. In an efficient kinetic link, energy in both the backswing and downswing moves from the lower body to the hips, trunk, shoulders, and out to the club. Read and reread this chapter. Once you have mastered the material, place yourself in various swing positions, such as the takeaway, top of the backswing, or impact. Pay attention to your ability to execute the swing. Determine where you are strong and stable or weak and lacking mobility.

Each chapter includes:

- 3D motion analysis—the newest technology in swing analysis—along with swing guru Hank Haney's experience and insights on the golf swing and swing faults.
- The physical cause of the swing fault, as explained by Hank Haney.
- The fitness solutions to the swing fault.

Further chapters outline the proper warm-up routine, how to build core strength, keys to a healthy back, and methods for improving posture, all of which provide you with a well-rounded golf fitness program.

You do not have to be Tiger Woods or an elite athlete to reap the benefits of a golf-specific fitness program. The body responds with the slightest amount of effort.

Three years ago a sixty-year-old devoted golfer walked into my studio, frustrated and feeling hopeless. Jim, who was recently retired, struggled with back pain. His physical therapist advised him to give up golf. For Jim that meant alienation from his social circle and the loss of the game that he passionately loved. Depression soon followed.

After a long discussion and a series of physical assessments I recommended that Jim undertake a short series of stretching and strengthening exercises for his back and hips. He committed to twenty minutes a day and within three months Jim was back on the course. My intention was not to make Jim's swing like Tiger's, Ernie's, or Vijay's. My intention was to have Jim play without pain and to return to the game he loved. If you're suffering from a common injury due to a swing flaw or a weakness in your musculoskeletal structure, *Swing Flaws and Fitness Fixes* can do the same for you.

Professional golfers have a team—a collaborative group of swing coaches, custom clubfitters, fitness trainers, sports psychologists, and nutritionists devoted to the athlete's peak performance. For the rest of us, *Swing Flaws and Fitness Fixes* is like having your own team of experts along with your PGA or LPGA instructor.

I am a lifelong golfer, a student of the golf swing, and a fitness expert with more than two decades of experience. I work with some of the best kinesiologists in the world, spend countless hours researching scientific studies on the swing, and perhaps most importantly, play and love the game. My intention for this book is to shift your old paradigm from frustration to hope and give you a renewed excitement for golf.

Together, Hank and I want to give you every opportunity for maximum performance on the course and a balanced, healthier life off the course.

In great golf and great health,

—KATHERINE

SWING FLAWS
AND
FITNESS FIXES

SECTION ONE

THE CONNECTION BETWEEN YOUR SWING AND FITNESS

CHAPTER ONE
WHY CONDITION
FOR GOLF?

EVERY GOLFER, AMATEUR or professional, wants to play better golf and lower his or her scores. Golf rules allow fourteen clubs in the bag, but there is actually a "fifteenth club": your body. Golf is often perceived as a game of technical skill rather than a sport that requires athleticism. This misperception usually results in mediocre performance and injury, because the golf swing is a very complex athletic movement. Golfers need to train the body just as an athlete would train for any other sport. To reach maximum potential the golfer must access all resources, blending instruction, technology, and the power of the body.

Tiger Woods and players of his generation have transformed the image of a golfer from that of a heavyset, cigar-smoking, potbellied hacker to a well-trained, physically powerful, talented athlete. You should look at golf the same way they do: as a *sport* played by *athletes*.

Even if you've never trained for golf, it's not too late to start. Fans of the Golf Channel often recognize me and stop me in airports for fitness advice. The encounter often goes like this: "Katherine, I love your work and I know I need to work on my flexibility, but I'm so inflexible that I don't know where to start." My response is usually, "Welcome to the club! Most golfers need to work on their flexibility. Regardless of your age or current fitness level you will reap the benefits of my golf-specific fitness program." Give yourself a break; this is a very difficult sport, especially if you take up the game later in life.

Over the past twenty years I have worked with thousands of golfers, some well into their nineties. The biggest determinant of success isn't how long you've been training, but rather how dedicated you are once you start. First determine your golf, fitness, and lifestyle goals, and then determine a realistic amount of time you are willing to devote to the program. Start with the basics and work your way up, but just make sure you keep at it.

To understand how important the right physical fitness program is to your golf game, just imagine a high-performance race car. It is a machine that requires specialized care, the right fuel, perfectly fitted parts, and ongoing maintenance. In the same way, it is critical that your golf fitness program be designed for the unique demands of the sport. Many golfers, for example, believe that cardio conditioning is important for endurance on the course, so they spend forty-five minutes a day on the treadmill, walking at a fast pace on one plane of intensity. They may feel like they're training for the sport, but in reality, they're not. I have played many, many golf courses and have never seen one that was completely flat and required monotonous exertion throughout the entire round. To say it a different way, playing a round of golf is nothing like walking on a treadmill! A complete golf fitness program requires all of the following:

- Flexibility
- Strength
- Core conditioning
- Balance
- Explosive/speed training
- Posture
- Mental focus
- Energy management
- Proper recovery

THE GOLFER AND INJURY

Injuries due to golf are most often associated with the repetitive stress of practice and play. During a typical round the golfer:

- Walks approximately 4–5 miles
- Makes more than a hundred practice and actual swings
- Leans over 30–40 putts
- Bends down 40–50 times

It's not surprising, then, that 30 percent of all professional golfers play injured, and that 53 percent of male and 45 percent of female golfers suffer from back pain.

When an athlete is injured, careful consideration must be given to the cause of the injury. Physical therapists and physicians often focus on removing the pain, usually with medication and rest, rather than addressing the root of the problem. But the problems usually continue once the golfer resumes playing. My program gives you the best chance to deal with injuries by prescribing exercise that can heal existing injuries and reduce the risk of developing new ones.

THE ROBERTS FLEX-FIT METHOD: THE NEXT EVOLUTION IN GOLF PERFORMANCE

Golf is the loneliest sport. You're completely alone with every conceivable opportunity to defeat yourself. Golf brings out your assets and liabilities as a person. The longer you play, the more certain you are that a man's performance is the outward manifestation of who, in his heart, he really thinks he is.

—HALE IRWIN

One thing I know for sure is that everything changes, including our bodies. What we strived for in our twenties changes in our thirties, forties, and so on. When I watch advertising for fitness products, I realize that they're targeting a very small demographic of our society, especially when you consider that by the year 2010,

50 percent of the U.S. population will be over the age of fifty. Rock-hard abs? Of course, who doesn't want rock-hard abs? But how about a fitness program designed to maximize our potential on the golf course? What about powerful posture and strong, flexible, lean bodies capable of sustaining us through life with energy, mental acuity, and a deep sense of overall wellness and purpose? How about a fitness program that teaches you ways to manage your energy, encourages times of rest and recovery, and facilitates muscular balance as well as a balanced life?

In my more than twenty years as a fitness professional, my students have run the gamut from juniors to seniors, the physically challenged to high-performance professional athletes. This experience as well as my own personal journey has led to the development of a unique golf performance program: The Roberts Flex-Fit Method.

One of the focuses of the Roberts Flex-Fit Method is muscular balance. The root cause of poor performance on the course and pain off the course is usually muscle imbalance. Due in large part to our sedentary lifestyle, we have developed imbalances of strength and flexibility in the body. Over time, the shortened muscles tug on the opposing muscles and cause weakness and wear. For example, in working with my students, I often find muscle imbalance in their hip flexors. Tight hip flexors weaken the opposing muscles, the glutes. Likewise, tight abdominals may cause a weakening of the back muscles. In my program we work the muscles of the front of the body and the back of the body together, and also balance flexibility and strength conditioning with periods of recovery. When possible we use compound movements, which enhance proprioception, the body's natural ability to control movement. Flexion exercises are balanced with extension, strength with flexibility, and balance with breath.

Every exercise in the Roberts Flex-Fit Method allows for modifications that can provide every golfer with the possibility for success. Based on the concept of building blocks, we present the fundamentals of the exercise, and once you're prepared, guide you from the basics to more advanced levels.

Basketball players, runners, swimmers, and divers, to name a few, are stronger and more powerful than ever. If we look at the scores or times posted in these sports, we can clearly see that athletes today are faster, more powerful, and have better training techniques at their disposal.

In golf we often look to technological advances to "save us." We think we can buy a better game. Let me make myself perfectly clear. Advances in technology are dramatic, and I firmly believe that critical elements to peak performance include custom-fitted clubs, the best and most appropriate type of ball, and apparel that protects and performs in all conditions. However, to purchase this technology without implementing a golf fitness program is like buying the high-performance race car and fueling it with mud.

Here are some shocking examples that show that even with improved club and ball technology, golf scores haven't come down that much over the years. In 1939, Ralph Guldahl won the Masters with a score of 279. Fifty-five years later, in 1994, José Maria Olazábal won the tournament with the same score. Dow Finsterwald won the 1958 PGA Championship with a score of 276. In 2005, Phil Mickelson took the title with an identical 276.

As Dr. Bob Rotella, author of *The Golf of Your Dreams*, notes, "Fifteen years ago the average American male golfer's handicap was 16.2. The average female golfer's handicap was 29. Today, the average American male golfer's handicap is 16.2, and the average female golfer's handicap is 29!" Clearly, golf handicaps have remained unchanged despite technological advances. In my opinion, golfers need to start accessing the most important club in their bag: their body.

CHAPTER TWO
ANATOMY OF THE GOLF SWING

When a golfer's muscles develop hardness and size like a weightlifter's, they retard the ease and quickness of hitting, which count so much at the instant of impact.

—HARRY VARDON

G OLF IS A physically demanding sport. A solid golf swing is a result of the upper body rotating around a solid, stable base—the lower body. Regardless of the efficiency of your swing, the biomechanics of the golf swing place a tremendous amount of stress on the body. To improve your game, you must have a basic understanding of these biomechanics and the muscles that are activated during various phases of the motion.

For our purposes, when we discuss muscular activity in the swing we are referring to professional or low-handicap, highly skilled, right-handed golfers. This is the baseline we use as the "standard" for muscle activity in the swing. However, I want to stress the importance of honoring your own body. I want to provide you with this information so you can more easily understand the golf swing. Just as every body has different levels of flexibility and strength, there are also many ways to swing the golf club.

This chapter of the book is perhaps the most important for you. My suggestion is to read the content and continually refer back to the information so you fully understand the biomechanics of the golf swing and the physiological correlations of the body and the swing. In this chapter I address the larger, overall muscle function of the golf swing as well as the smaller, more specific movements. If this information is new to you, focus on the general understanding of the golf swing. If you are well versed in the biomechanics of the swing, you will find the expanded content to be very informative.

TYPES OF GOLF SWINGS

The classic golf swing, exemplified by Bobby Jones, incorporated a large body turn, with an equal amount of hip and shoulder rotation in the backswing. We estimate the hip turn to be between 70 and 80 degrees. Typically this swing created a flatter swing plane. The finish position shows the hips facing the target, shoulders turned beyond the target and the spine in a neutral, upright, balanced, and relaxed finish position.

In contrast, the modern golf swing, exemplified in the past by Jack Nicklaus and today by players such as Tiger Woods, incorporates a steeper swing plane and a large shoulder turn and torso rotation over a more stable lower body. This limited hip rotation, at approximately 45 degrees, features less lower-body rotation than the classic swing—it instead creates resistance through the coiling action of the spine and the shoulders. This action creates the foundation from which the torso rotates around the hips, and we thus see a greater hip-to-shoulder ratio of turn.

Over the past few years various golf instructors have identified other "types" of golf swings. Whether you use a one-plane or two-plane swing, or the newest style, the stack and tilt, or a classic or modern swing, understanding how the body works in the various phases of the swing will help you understand your swing flaws and the best method for treating those flaws.

THE KINEMATIC SEQUENCE—
UNDERSTANDING AN EFFICIENT GOLF SWING

Nobody asked how you looked, just what you shot.

—SAM SNEAD

The golf industry invests millions in the development of new technological advances. I believe in the power of technology and feel we should use every available tool to make us better golfers. In the past the naked eye and video analysis were the sole methods of capturing the golf swing and giving us feedback. Fortunately, we now have the use of 3D motion analysis, which enables us to measure much more than two-dimensional video ever could. We can now capture what's called the "kinematic sequence" of the golf swing.

The kinematic sequence is a measure of how the golfer generates speed in the body and how efficiently the golfer transfers energy from various parts of the body to the clubhead. The sequence begins in the lower body and pelvis, travels to the trunk and shoulders, then to the arms, and then out to the clubhead at the top of the backswing. Imagine a car race. Which car hits the finish line first? Which car slams into the wall? In the golf swing, the lower body comes in first during the backswing, the torso in second, the shoulders in third, the arms in fourth, and the clubhead last. As the golfer begins the downswing the exact same sequence needs to occur for an efficient swing. The lower body gets the checkered flag, followed by the trunk and shoulders, the arms, and then the clubhead. If one part of your body "slams into the wall," the entire body or field of cars is in danger of not finishing the swing. Swing flaws occur when this order of sequencing is inefficient. Proper sequencing is primary to efficient ballstriking and is the key to accuracy. Many golfers have different ways of getting the clubhead square at impact—take a look at the swings of Jim Furyk and Ernie Els—but the best golfers have nearly identical kinematic sequences.

An efficient kinematic sequence involves not just acceleration, but deceleration. In fact, deceleration is just as, if not more, important than acceleration, because it is essential for the transference of energy. This is how we harness power and generate maximum velocity at impact. Envision a wet dish towel. As you coil the towel in your hand you are creating energy. When you "snap" the towel, explosive power occurs and is the result of not only the acceleration but deceleration of energy. This acceleration/deceleration relationship represents what occurs in an efficient kinematic sequence when the phases of the golfer's body follows the proper sequence. Tour players not only harness their energy with an efficient coiling of the body, but they efficiently decelerate and utilize their power by harnessing their energy in the downswing. Golfers who hit the ball long off the tee activate their lower body before they have fully reached their optimal coil in the backswing. Their hips decelerate while their upper body continues to accelerate.

The Arc of the Sequence

When reading the kinematic sequence graph we look at the arc of the body's action. A spike in the arc represents acceleration, or speed, while the decline in the arc represents deceleration, or the power generated by the golfer. The steeper the curve of the arc, the more acceleration; the flatter the arc, the less deceleration. In a nutshell, speed and energy transfer at the point of deceleration.

Below is an example of an efficient kinematic sequence. The vertical line represents the point of impact. Notice how the arms have started to decelerate at the point of impact.

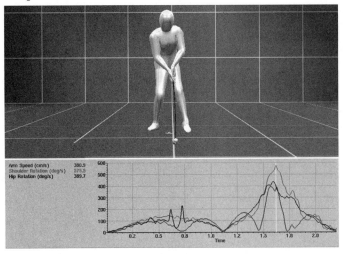

This graph is an example of an efficient kinematic sequence. Notice the arc of the hips, shoulders, and arms are all at their maximum point of acceleration and deceleration at impact, representing a proper sequence.

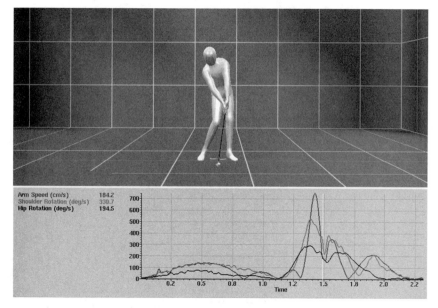

Arm Speed (cm/s)	184.2
Shoulder Rotation (deg/s)	330.7
Hip Rotation (deg/s)	194.5

This is going to deliver sluggish clubhead speed, and it explains why the shoulder speed is so high at impact. The sluggish feel leads to a subconscious attempt to muscle through with an artificial acceleration or pull-through response. There is no cracking of the towel here.

Compared side by side, you can see the golfer on the right has the majority of his weight on the right leg at impact, which causes the aforementioned lift-and-pull-through action. Note: the dotted line represents an inefficient sequence.

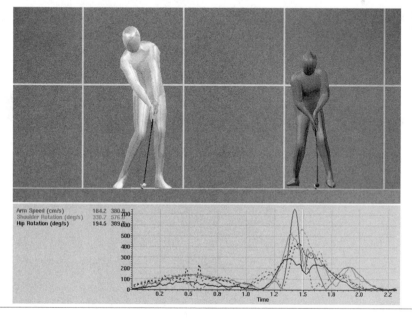

Arm Speed (cm/s)	184.2	380.9
Shoulder Rotation (deg/s)	330.7	576.0
Hip Rotation (deg/s)	194.5	389.0

SPINE ANATOMY

For golfers, proper spine function is essential to the efficient activation of the coiling and uncoiling of the spine that is needed to produce a powerful swing. The spine has a natural S-shape, which is referred to as the "neutral" position. This angle must be maintained to protect the spine while playing golf. There are seven vertebrae in the neck (cervical), twelve vertebrae in the mid-back (thoracic) and five vertebrae in the lower back (lumbar). Below the lumbar spine we find the sacrum and coccyx bones.

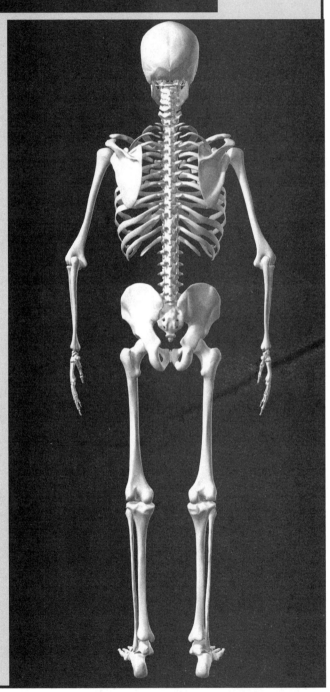

MUSCLES OF THE BODY

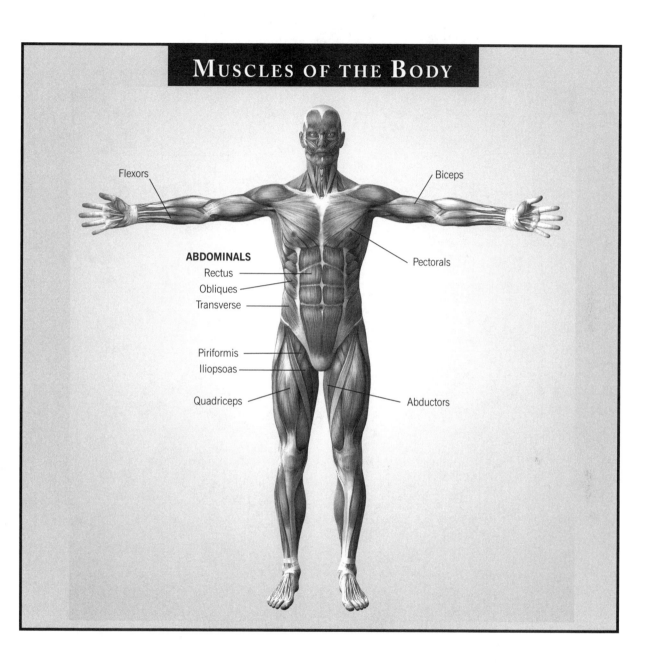

Flexors

Biceps

ABDOMINALS

Rectus

Obliques

Transverse

Pectorals

Piriformis

Iliopsoas

Quadriceps

Abductors

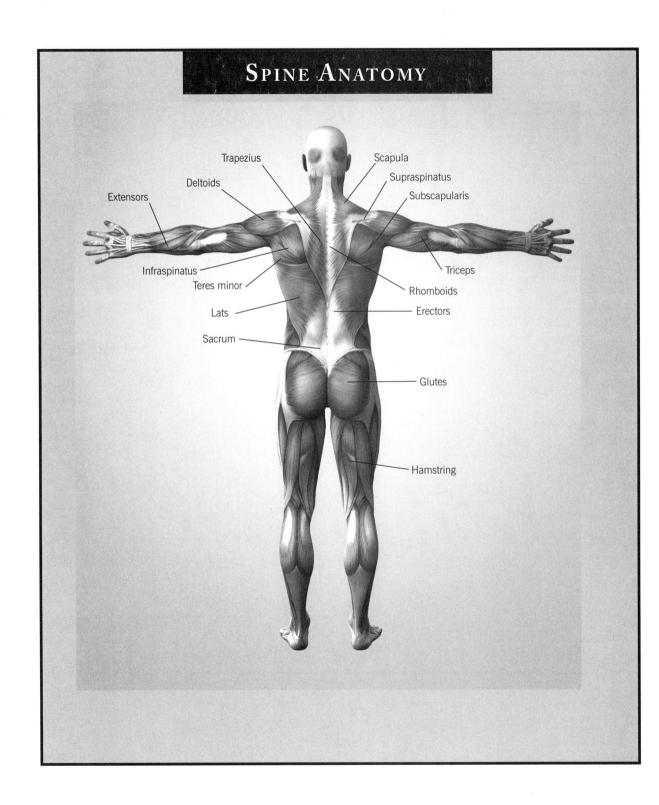

SPINE ANATOMY

Extensors

Trapezius

Deltoids

Scapula

Supraspinatus

Subscapularis

Infraspinatus

Teres minor

Triceps

Rhomboids

Lats

Erectors

Sacrum

Glutes

Hamstring

TYPES OF MUSCLE ACTIVITY

Throughout this book I describe various muscle activities in various phases of the golf swing and during the exercises. When I use terms such as "activate," "engage," and "contract," I am referring to the contraction of the muscle being discussed. Let's discuss types of muscle activity. Think about doing a bicep curl. As you bend your elbow and bring the weight toward your shoulder, the bicep is in a concentric or shortened state. At the same time the opposing muscle, the tricep, is in an eccentric or lengthened state of activity. Isometric or static tension is contraction of the muscle without joint movement. Imagine that your palms are pressing together in front of your chest, activating your pec muscles. This is an example of an isometric activity.

PHASES OF THE SWING

The following is a description of "normal" anatomy and biomechanics during the golf swing. Use this information as your guide, identifying the muscle groups activated during specific phases of your swing. This information will help you identify your strengths and weaknesses and let you develop a tailored fitness program.

There are six phases of the golf swing:

- Address
- Takeaway: Includes early and late backswing
- Top of the backswing
- Downswing: Includes acceleration
- Impact
- Follow-through: Includes early follow-through and full finish position

Address

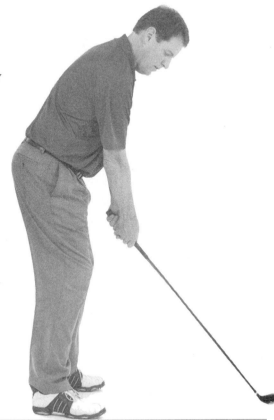

The address is the static position of your body just prior to initiating the golf swing.

The upper body leans forward, allowing the clubhead to come in contact with the ground. The golfer should bend forward from the hips and keep the spine in a neutral, upright posture, without an excessive arch in the lower spine or a rounded mid-back. This spine position, combined with the natural relaxed position of the shoulders and arms, is called the "neutral" position. At address, the center of gravity and weight distribution is over the middle of the feet. The muscles of the hips, trunk, and neck are active. A slight bend in the knees activates the hamstrings, which are the muscles at the back of the thighs. The arms, forearms, wrists, and hands show slight activation. Some of the major lower extremity muscles are also active and functioning as stabilizers. These muscles include the quadriceps, groin, the Achilles tendons, and the feet.

Takeaway or Early Backswing, Late Backswing, and Top of the Backswing

The takeaway or early backswing phase defines the position you're in as you begin to draw back the club to initiate the backswing.

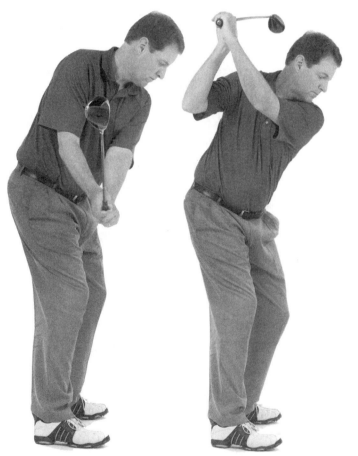

The late backswing is the position in which the wrist is hinged and the shaft of the club is perpendicular to the ground. It is between the early backswing, or when the hands have moved past the right leg but not yet reached the height of the shoulders, and the top of the backswing, when your hands have moved to a position just opposite or slightly higher than the top of the shoulders and the clubshaft is parallel to the ground.

This phase has the club at its highest point, right before the downswing begins.

The takeaway is activated by the trunk and abdominal muscles. These muscles stabilize the spine from the top of the pelvis to the bottom of the ribs. The back and abdominal muscles, specifically on the left side, are activated, protecting you from injury. Additionally the left shoulder and quad muscle of the right leg are activated. As the club moves away from the ball the most active muscles are the upper and middle traps, left side muscles of the back, and abdominal oblique.

During the takeaway, approximately 75 percent of your weight transfers to the right leg. The trunk, arms, and pelvis begin to rotate, and the initial process of coiling around the axis of the spine begins. At this point we begin to feel the connection between the spine and right hip. The shoulder and chest muscles are active as the club moves away from the ball.

At the top of the backswing we see a difference in the amount of rotation in the shoulders and hips. For touring professionals we often see a 45-degree hip turn and a 90-degree shoulder rotation. The differential between these motions is called the "X-factor." Originally introduced by Jim McLean in 1992, the X-factor refers to the stretch in the torso as a result of the difference between the rotation of the shoulders and the rotation of the hips during the golf swing. Research proves that longer drives can be directly attributed to the differential between shoulder and hip rotation. Although increasing your X-factor has been shown to increase distance, golfers will see greater benefits from working within their physical capabilities rather than trying to move beyond their range of motion.

The muscles of the legs and right hip are contracted. Specifically, the right hip rotates internally while the left hip rotates externally. In Tour players we see the lower body, specifically the right glute, become engaged and start the downswing before the player reaches the full backswing. This coiling in different directions generates power, but it can also cause injury.

Side-bending describes the amount of sway that occurs as the golfer moves into the backswing. Excessive side-bending causes the left shoulder and head to dip at the top of the backswing, causing a reverse pivot that places extreme stress on the low back.

The right hip internal rotators and left hip external rotators are contracted. The oblique abdominals, lats, and the spinal erector muscles rotate the trunk and are extremely active at the top of the backswing.

The golfer's weight shifts to the inner part of the right foot.

The hands, wrists, and forearms are activated to control the weight and direction of the club.

Downswing and Acceleration

In this phase the club is brought from the top of the backswing toward impact.

Acceleration refers to the transition of the downswing moments before impact.

For golfers, the proper sequence transfers motion first from the lower body to the torso, then through the shoulders and hands, and finally to the club, maximizing speed at ball impact. It is essential for the muscles of the trunk, the abdominal erectors, and the glutes to be active during this phase. This muscle activity will ensure stability for the back. The transition at the top of backswing occurs when the swing changes direction and "uncoils." This is the most physically active phase of the golf swing. The highest forces of side-bending, shear, and rotation occur at the neck and lower back during this phase. Additionally, the left rhomboids and traps are active, as well as the right-side chest muscles. In the lower body the right glute is 100 percent activated, followed by the quad and adductor muscles.

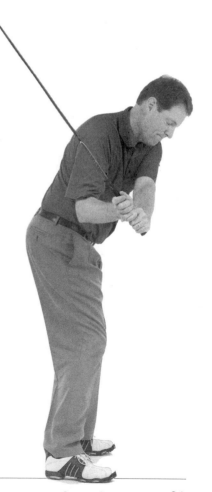

In highly skilled golfers the lower body, specifically the hips, slows down before the golfer reaches the top of the backswing and the hips change direction. The hips are now rotating toward the target while the upper body continues to coil in the backswing. In the downswing the lower body initiates the movement. The lower body, specifically the hips, has a higher rate of velocity than the upper body, so power in the swing is primarily generated from the hips and lower body. In addition to the hips, the left hamstring, glute, and quad are active. On the right side the oblique is most active, followed by the right glute.

The acceleration phase of the swing refers to the time between the transition from the backswing to the downswing until just before impact. In addition to the lower body activity, the chest muscles, or pecs, are contracted at this time. On the right side, the second-most active muscle is the upper serratus (anterior); on the left side it is the levator scapulae.

A Word on Wrist Hinge in the Downswing

The wrist hinge position in your downswing helps you harness energy. As the arms move in the downswing, the angle of the wrist to the forearm becomes smaller and then begins to widen at impact. The correct wrist angle is critical because it creates lag and load in the downswing. When the wrists unhinge at the correct moment, clubhead speed increases. During this "wrist lag action" in the downswing—in which the right elbow reaches the right hip and the hands come to waist height—the hands begin to release as the clubshaft moves toward the ball. The wrists unhinge after impact and the forearms pronate and supinate from the backswing position and release toward the target. When we lose this angle at the wrist, swing flaws such as casting and scooping occur.

Impact

The phase of the golf swing during which the club makes contact with the ball.

At the point of impact practically

every muscle and joint in the body is moving. At impact we strive for maximum club-head speed, which creates maximum velocity when contact is made with the ball.

The mid- and lower back experience a side-bending motion toward the right combined with a rotational motion toward the left. The lower body is turning, and the hips are slightly open toward the target. The shoulders are brought back to a square position, with the entire shoulder girdle working. Specifically, the shoulders, rotators, and mid-back shoulder-stabilizer muscles are active, to help generate speed at impact. The trunk muscles, abdominals, and the erector spinae are also active.

The muscles of the hips, adductors, abductors, and legs are active. Specifically, the right hip rotates externally while the left hip rotates internally. External rotation refers to the turning of the thigh or pelvis outward, away from the center of the body. Internal rotation refers to the turning of the thigh or pelvis inward, toward the center of the body.

The head and neck experience a side-bending motion toward the right, combined with a forward bend. Flexion and pronation of the right forearm occurs through impact.

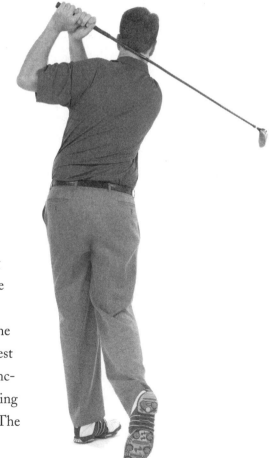

Finish and Early Follow-Through

The early follow-through is defined as the point immediately after impact. The finish position is defined as the end of the golf swing after impact, when the club is horizontal to the ground.

In the early follow-through phase of the swing the trunk begins to decelerate. The chest or pec muscles are active. The lower-body function is similar to impact, with the left hamstring and quad acting as the stabilizing foundation. The right glute remains active, as well as the abdominal and trunk-stabilizing muscles. In the early follow-through, just past impact, the left forearm supinates and the right forearm pronates.

The finish position is a full extension of the body toward the target. The club is horizontal to the ground at the end of the swing. With the spine in a straight position, the finish usually generates minimal stress on the body, unless the golfer presents with a hyperextended spine. This excessive bending or arching of the spine can cause injury to the back.

The hips and trunk turn toward the target. The left hip rotates, straightens, and moves toward the midline of the body, while the right hip moves to a "neutral" position facing the target. The left knee straightens, supported by the left hamstring, quad, and adductor, while the right quad is active. The right knee remains bent, with balance on the toes.

The spine maintains a "neutral" or slightly side-bent position toward the right. The shoulders are active, specifically the left shoulder and the pec, as well as the shoulder-stabilizing muscles. The arms supinate toward the target.

UNDERSTANDING POSTURE

For our purposes we can think of posture as "the position from which movement begins and ends." This definition is particularly useful when you consider that a person's posture is a physical result of the interaction between his or her body, nervous system, and musculoskeletal system.

Static Posture

Static posture is the position of the body without movement (for example, the address position).

Dynamic Posture

Dynamic posture describes the axis of the spine during movement. One definition refers to dynamic posture as "the instantaneous axis of rotation of any/all working joints in any spatial or temporal relationship." If the joints are properly aligned, their ability to rotate around the axis occurs with minimal effort. This is important for the golf swing because many swing flaws occur when the spine is not able to rotate with a full range of motion.

Standing Posture

Standing posture is defined as the position in which the ankles, hips, trunk, and head are aligned vertically and the curvatures of the spine are optimal. This can also be defined as static, because you are not moving, but we use this standing posture to evaluate misalignment in your posture. Check your posture in the mirror from the side and front views.

CHAPTER THREE
PHYSICAL ASSESSMENTS
AND GUIDELINES
FOR SUCCESS

Golf is said to be a humbling game, but it is surprising how many people
are either not aware of their weaknesses or else reckless of consequences.

—BOBBY JONES

YOU NEED TO know where you have been to know where you need to go, and thus my program starts with baseline physical assessments. Once you understand your flexibility, strength, and stability challenges, you'll be better equipped to formulate a plan of action.

Methods for testing:

1. Take a golf lesson. If you have access to a PGA/LPGA instructor, have your swing videotaped and swing-analyzed by a professional. Tell the instructor you are beginning a golf-specific fitness program. Share your golf and fitness goals with the instructor. I believe this is worth the investment, because their insight is invaluable and it gives you a baseline from which you can chart your results. If they have a launch monitor, have your clubhead speed checked as well.

2. Use a buddy. Ask a friend to assist you with the physical assessments. Have them administer your assessments and chart your mobility, stability, strength, and

balance results. Using a friend allows you to focus on the test and not on charting the results.

3. Use a mirror. If you are by yourself, estimate the angles of mobility by using a mirror. Time yourself when necessary and write down the results.

When you perform the tests below, keep a log of the results: Rate the difficulty of each test on a scale from one to five, and also chart your angles of mobility. The photos provide you with an estimation of angles of mobility. You should retest yourself every four weeks and take new measurements.

STANDING TESTS

Standing Baseline Rotation Test

Stand with your feet hip-width apart. Inhale as you lift your right arm to shoulder height. Exhale as you rotate the upper body around to the right. Line up the forefinger with a stationary spot on the wall or ceiling behind you. Remember that spot and switch sides.

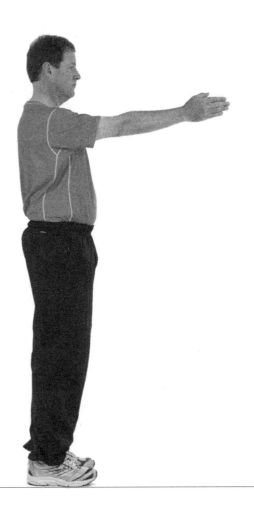

Standing Pelvic Tilt Test

Stand in your address position with your arms crossed over your chest. Without moving your upper body, create an arch in your lumbar spine. Tuck your pelvis under and return to the starting position, or neutral spine. Determine your mobility in each direction. For example, is it easier for you to arch your back or tuck your pelvis under? Do you experience any shaking in the body in either direction? The goal is to have equal mobility in the hips in each direction. Chart the range of motion in the hips. Note: Placing a golf club along your spine in the starting, neutral position helps you see if you have an arch in your lower back.

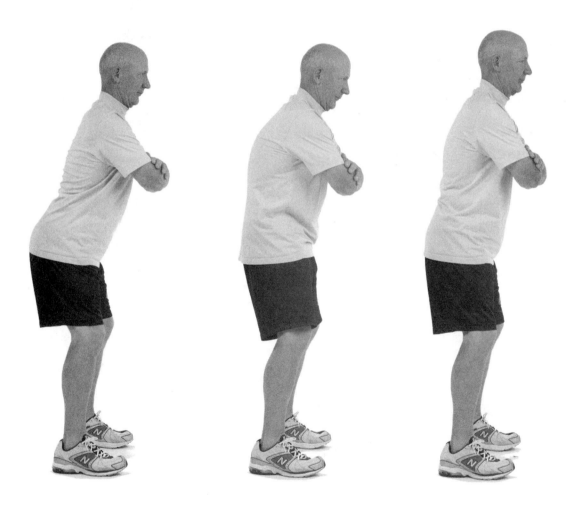

Standing Hamstring Mobility Test with Chair

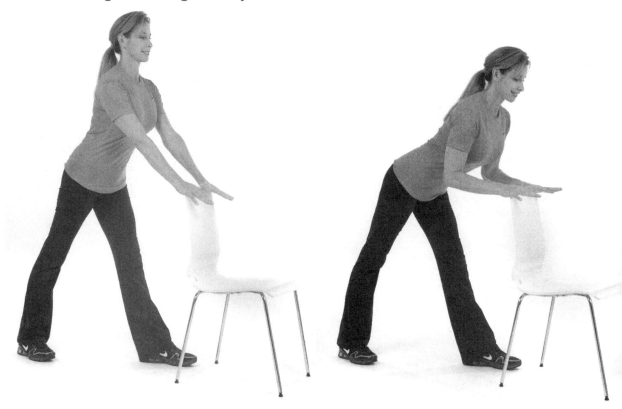

This test is primarily for hamstring flexibility but will also test hip and back mobility. From your address position, step your right foot back, internally rotating your right leg and foot at a 45-degree angle. Place your hands on the back of a chair and hinge from your hips, bringing your upper body forward as far as possible and feeling the stretch in the left hamstring. Determine how far forward you need to bend before you feel the stretch in your hamstrings. Switch sides and repeat.

Standing Wall Lat Test

This tests the mobility of your shoulders and large muscles of the trunk, the lats. Place your back against a wall, knees bent at a 90-degree angle, and lift your right arm above your head. Try to touch your thumb to the wall behind you. Measure the angle of your upper arm to the wall. Switch sides and repeat. Note: Maintain a connection between your lower back and the wall.

Single-Leg Balance Test

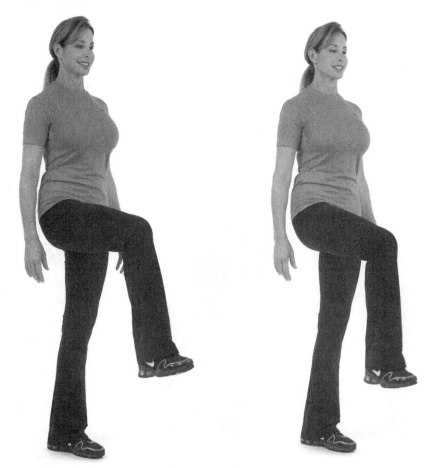

Shift your weight onto your left leg and lift your right leg off the floor. Hold for as long as possible and record the time you are able to balance. Close the eyes and retest. Repeat with your other leg. Lifting your right leg measures the stability of your left leg. Note: Keep in mind that any past injuries to the feet, ankles, or hips may alter the test results.

Standing Pelvic Rotation, Trunk Mobility, and Coordination Test

This tests lower-body mobility, upper-body mobility, and the ability to rotate the upper and lower body separately; it also coordinates all of the components of the swing in one movement. Stand in your address position with your arms crossed over your chest.

Without moving your upper body, internally and externally rotate the hips only.

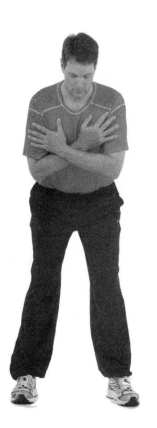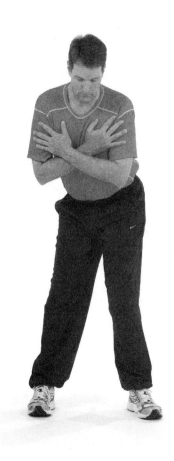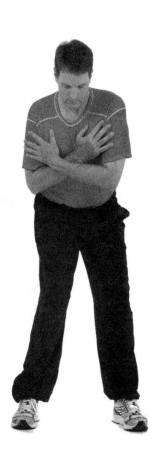

First revolve the right hip inward and the left hip out. Then revolve the left hip inward as the right hip revolves outward. Isolate the hip movement **without** moving your torso or shoulders.

Now keep your hips still and rotate your torso and shoulders **only,** estimating the range of motion in your trunk, mid-back, and shoulders.

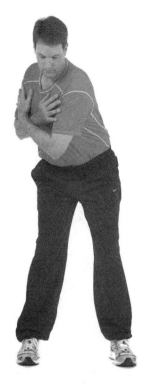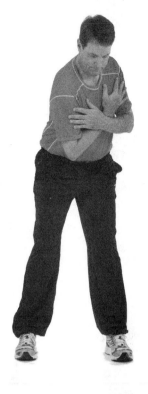

Now rotate your hips, torso, and shoulders together as if you were approaching the top of the backswing. Initiate the down-swing from your hips, with your torso and shoulders coming into a full finish position. Are you able to coordinate your move-ment with the hips leading the backswing and downswing?

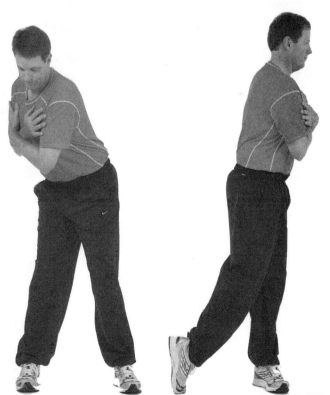

Standing Shoulder Mobility Test

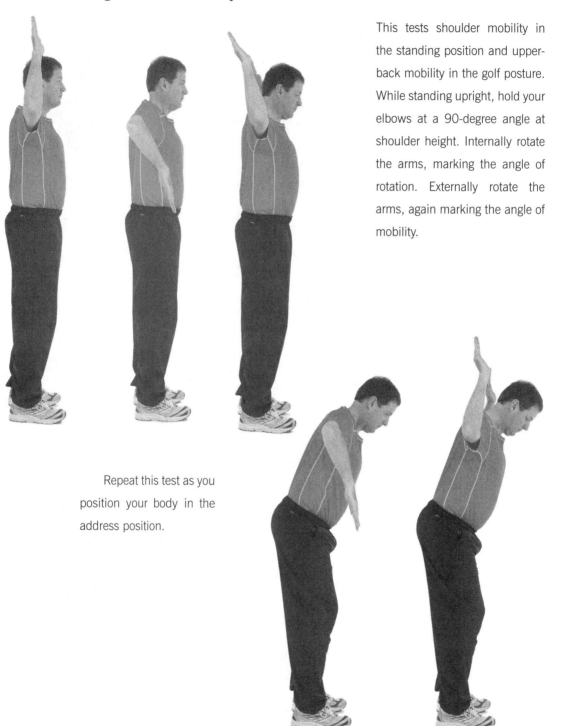

This tests shoulder mobility in the standing position and upper-back mobility in the golf posture. While standing upright, hold your elbows at a 90-degree angle at shoulder height. Internally rotate the arms, marking the angle of rotation. Externally rotate the arms, again marking the angle of mobility.

Repeat this test as you position your body in the address position.

SEATED TESTS

Seated Wall Test

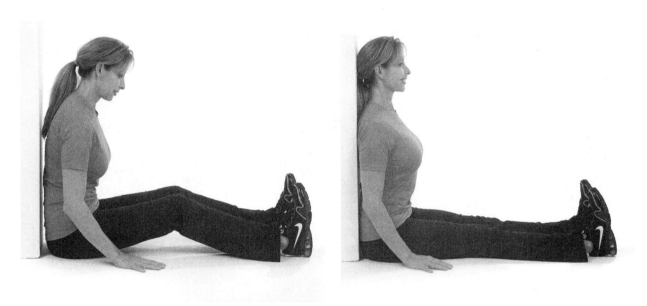

This tests hamstring and upper-back mobility. Sit with your back against the wall and extend your legs, pressing your knees toward the floor. Sit up as tall as possible and squeeze your shoulder blades together, bringing your head to the wall. Measure the distance between the backs of your knees and the floor. Measure the distance required to place your shoulders against the wall.

Lunge Trunk Rotation/Hip Stabilization Test

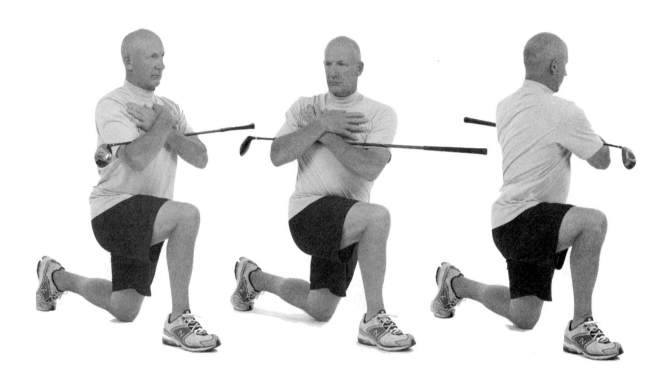

This tests trunk mobility and hip/adductor strength, along with the ability to rotate the upper body separately from the lower body. Place your left knee on the floor, with your right leg bent at a 90-degree angle. Try to place your knee and foot in one line. Place a club across your chest and stabilize your hips. Rotate your upper body to the right and the left without moving the hips. Move slowly, measuring your trunk flexibility. Pay attention to the point in your trunk rotation at which the hips begin to lose stability. Measure your range of motion and ability to stabilize the hips on the right and left side. Switch legs and repeat test.

PRONE TESTING

Hip Flexor Mobility

This tests flexibility in the psoas/hip flexors. Lying on your back in a supine position, bring your knees to your chest. Keep your left knee lifted placing your hands around your left knee as you allow your right leg to fall toward the floor. Measure the distance between your hamstring and the ground. Switch legs and repeat.

Supine Hip Internal/External Mobility Test

This tests your internal and external hip mobility. While lying on your back, bring your knees up with your fists placed between the knees. Internally and externally rotate the legs. Measure the mobility in the hips, paying attention to the differences in each hip and in each direction. Note: Go back to the standing pelvic rotation test. Are the results of this test consistent with the results of the previous test?

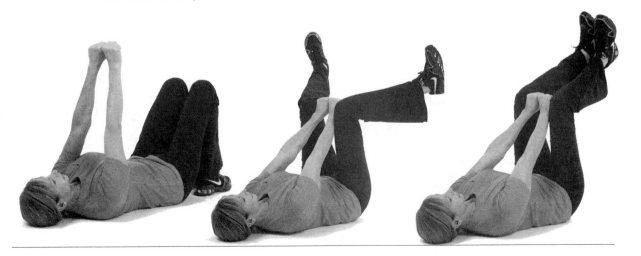

Bridge Pose Test

This tests your glute strength and your ability to activate your right and left glutes separately. While lying on your back, lift your hips off the floor as high as possible. Measure how long you can hold this position

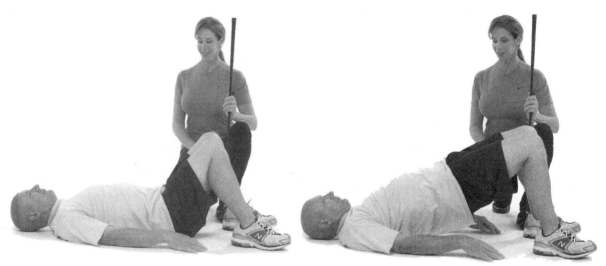

Bridge Pose Test with One Leg Extended

Place a club across your hips. With the club balanced on the hips, extend one leg, hold for thirty seconds, and switch sides. Measure your ability to extend your leg without the club sliding or without one hip falling below the other hip.

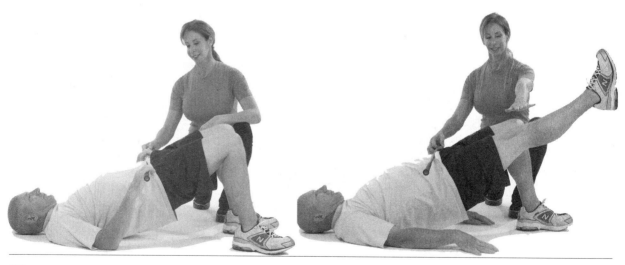

Spinal/Hip Disassociation Test

Tests lumbar and thoracic spine mobility. Lie on your side and bring your knees to a 90-degree angle while you rest on your right shoulder. Note: Support your head and neck with a towel. Bring the arms to shoulder height, palms together. Maintain a connection between the knees. Inhale deeply, and as you exhale, roll the upper body open, bringing the left arm as close to the floor as possible. Measure the distance of your left shoulder to the floor and measure the point at which your back immobility causes your knees to separate. Switch sides and repeat.

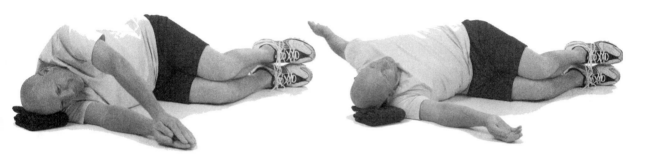

GUIDELINES FOR SUCCESS:

- *Obtain written permission from your physician before participating in this or any other physical fitness program.*
- Find a quiet place, free from interruptions and loud noises. The space should be warm to ensure that muscles remain flexible.
- Set goals and be realistic. Adherence to the program is more important than completing as many exercises as possible.
- You should never experience pain, either in the muscles, joints, or nerves. Slight discomfort as the muscle is stretching is acceptable, but pain is not. Be gentle and patient—Rome wasn't built in a day.
- Always modify the exercise, paying keen attention to your body's reaction.
- Never "bounce" in a stretch or use momentum when working on strength. Bouncing or "ballistic" stretching may cause injury.
- Remember to flex the opposing muscle. This will create a stretch reflex in the antagonist muscle, sending the message for the muscle to relax. For example,

it is necessary to squeeze, flex, or engage the quadriceps when attempting to stretch the hamstring.

- It is always helpful to keep the "core" slightly engaged. That refers to gently "drawing the navel toward the spine" at all times. This facilitates support of the lumbar spine. In addition, lifting the rib cage off the waist supports better posture and increases diaphragmatic breathing capacity.
- Have fun!

CHAPTER FOUR
ACCESSING YOUR UNTAPPED POWER SOURCE—BREATHING

One thing a golfer has to learn is that it is not the game he played last year, or last week, or probably will play the week after next, that he commands in any one event. He has only his game at the time; and it may be far from his best—but it's all he has, and he'd just as well harden his heart and make the most of it.

—WALTER HAGEN

I do know that when you are free of tension you can swing faster, and that definitely is a good thing.

—HANK HANEY

IN MY HOME the Golf Channel is on constantly. I love watching golf for many reasons: seeing great shots that inspire me, appreciating the talent of the Tour players, and listening to the commentators. I've noticed that the announcers always talk about the keen mental focus of the players, their ability to stay in the moment, and the way the players control their emotions. When I travel as a teacher

I always ask my students what is it they are looking to gain from my session with them, and many say they want to learn how to focus their minds. In a recent issue of a golf magazine, a reader's poll conducted a survey in which 87 percent of the readers agreed that golf is a mental game but only 2 percent said they would seek out a sports psychologist for advice. If you want to focus your mind you have to get serious about it, and you should start by developing an awareness of your breathing. With practice you can use your breathing to quiet your mind.

First-tee jitters, hitting over water, or swinging the club when an instructor is evaluating your swing is stressful. When Hank and I teach together I walk the practice tee assessing our students for physical restrictions and biomechanical flaws. My goal is to evaluate the golfer's swing and look for mechanical strengths and weaknesses. One of the most common swing flaws I see in our students is tension in their body (usually when Hank is about to evaluate their swing). This tension is typically a result of performance anxiety that stems from an overactive mind. Let's be honest here: Golf is mentally challenging, and an overactive mind has a direct effect on your physical performance.

Golf is a sport that requires a connection of body and mind. Compromised strength in the body stresses the mind, and vice versa. Your breathing pattern is the mirror of your internal physical and mental state. When Zach Johnson talked about his Masters win he described his state of mind as "very peaceful, a zone-like state." When the body is relaxed, the lungs, diaphragm, and muscles of the rib cage and chest move in an unrestricted way. But any time we experience stress on the golf course, our breathing becomes erratic. The physiological effect of holding the breath is a "fight or flight" response that stresses the entire nervous system. The result is rapid, uncontrolled breathing and a loss of blood flow to the extremities, including the brain. The body becomes tense, the mind races, and the ability to execute the golf swing becomes more challenging. (As if we need more challenge!)

POSTURE AND PROPER BREATHING

Diaphragmatic breathing, the expansion and contraction of the diaphragm, is the cure for reducing tension in the body and the most effective way to quiet the mind.

- Deep breathing supports proper blood flow to the entire body, relieving tension in the muscles that inhibit movement.
- Breathing enables you to quiet the mind and move into "the Zone."
- Proper breathing supports your energy level throughout the round.

When we over- or under-ventilate we reduce the oxygenation of the cells, causing muscle tension and physical and mental fatigue. The most effective way to breathe deeper is to elongate the spine. When we "slouch" we inhibit the function of the diaphragm. Ancient practices of movement such as yoga, tai chi, and many martial arts preach that breath begins from the base of the spine. One way we can access this power is through a methodology I call N.T.R. The navel (N) moves toward the spine, the tailbone (T) slightly tucks under, and the rib cage (R) lifts off the waist. The best way to practice this is from a standing position. Stand with your feet hip-width apart and place your palm slightly below your navel. Inhale as you press your navel toward your spine and slightly tuck your tailbone. Place your hands on your rib cage and on your exhale feel as if you are lifting your rib cage off your waist. Roll your shoulder blades together and down your back. Hold this powerful posture position for one minute, relax, and repeat five times. Eventually this strong posture position will become second nature.

Breathing and Your Pre-shot Routine

When and how do you breathe during your golf swing? The majority of golfers are not aware of their breathing patterns. Incorporating diaphragmatic breathing into your pre-shot routine will calm the mind and increase the sense of rhythm and tempo into your swing. Breathe in and out through the nose, which calms the nervous system. For higher-handicap golfers, begin by setting your stance, take a long slow deep breath in and out through the nose, and then begin your takeaway.

Paul Trittler, a *Golf Magazine* Top 100 Teacher and the Director of Instruction at the Kostis McCord Learning Center, offers advice for lower-handicap golfers. "As you stand behind the ball visualizing the ball flight, incorporate long, slow, deep breathing. As you sole the club, aim the face, set your back foot, and begin a deep inhalation. Then set your front foot, let your eyes go to the target and begin to exhale. Once you feel balanced and solid in your stance, complete your exhale. Allow your eyes to go to the ball and begin your swing."

The following exercises will help you develop diaphragmatic breathing. Practice these exercises every day.

Breathing Awareness Exercise

While lying on your back, place your fingertips gently on your rib cage. Slowly inhale through your nose for a count of four, and then exhale for a count of four. Focus on expanding and contracting your rib cage. Repeat ten to twenty times. When you feel you have mastered this breathing, extend the exhalation to a count of six. Repeat ten times.

Extended Side Stretch

Place your left hand, knee, and right foot in a straight line. Press your foot into the floor and pull your navel toward your spine. Inhale deeply and stretch

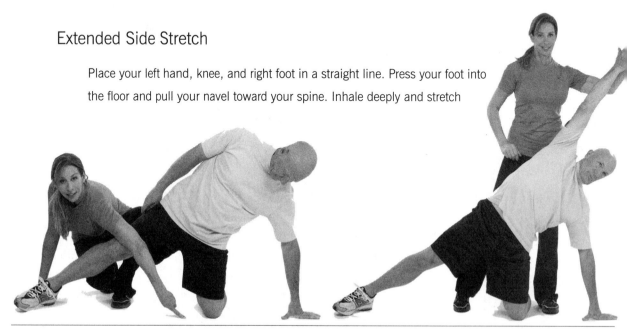

your right arm over your head. Hold for five to seven deep breaths and switch sides. The more you tuck your pelvis under (also known as creating a posterior tilt in your pelvis), the more you'll feel the stretch.

Supine Chest Stretch on the Ball

Roll a stability ball behind your upper spine, supporting your head. Lift your hips and engage your glutes until your lower body is parallel to the floor. Your arms should be at a 90-degree angle, pressing away from the ceiling toward the floor. Focus on the stretch in the chest and rib cage. Hold this position for ten deep breaths, inhaling and exhaling through the nose.

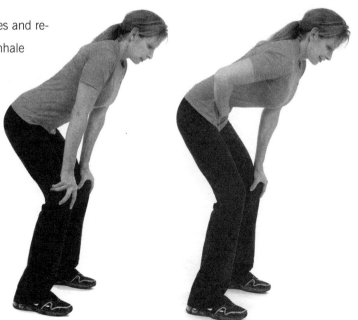

TVA Abdominal Lift

Place your hands on your knees and remove any arch in your back. Inhale deeply and exhale all the air out of your lungs. Hold the air out and sharply pull your navel into your spine. Hold for three seconds, release the TVAs (the lower abdominals) and inhale deeply again. Take five normal breaths and repeat five times. Note: Keep your head above your heart.

Passive Supine Chest Expansion

Lie down with a rolled-up towel under the length of your spine, from the base to your head. Your knees should be bent and your palms facing up. Relax in this position while you practice ten to twenty diaphragmatic breaths. As a variation, you can extend your legs and place the rolled-up towel under your knees.

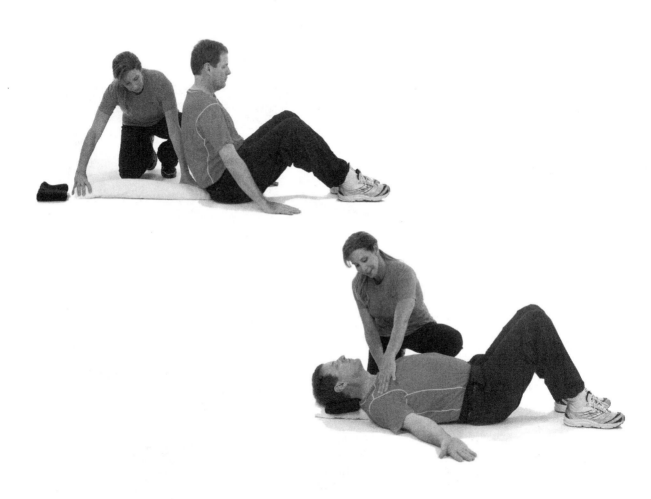

CHAPTER FIVE
PREPARING YOUR BODY WITH A WARM-UP FOR BODY AND MIND

Golf requires a lot of practice—a whole lot, in fact. I have practiced . . . six and seven hours at a stretch and all with one club. That is why when I am about to make a shot I know exactly what I can do with the club I am about to use. I know whether I can stop the ball two feet from the pin at a certain distance, because practice has taught me just how much effort I must use to accomplish the end I seek. I am sure of every shot I make.

—GENE SARAZEN

The purpose of a proper warm-up is to warm up the body, swing, and stroke, and to create confidence.

—PIA NILSSON AND LYNN MARRIOTT

THINK ABOUT HOW much time you spend getting ready before a round. Maybe you take aspirin, grab some tape for your fingers, the proper attire for the weather that day, and pack your bag with golf balls and tees. But do you prepare your body by stretching your golf-specific muscles? Do you find yourself "not warmed up" until the third, fourth, or fifth hole of your round? One component of golf fitness that is the easiest to practice and the most commonly overlooked is simply warming up for your round.

Here are a few thoughts from Hank Haney regarding the importance of a pre-round warm-up:

"Even if you are Tiger Woods and you are the best-conditioned golfer in the world, you still need to warm up before every round of golf. Going through a proper warm-up is one of the most overlooked parts of any golfer's day. If a player doesn't stretch and loosen up his or her body before they practice or play, they're risking injury. On top of that, chances are good that the player won't get their round off to a very good start because it usually means that they don't really get loosened up until about the sixth hole. Touring pros always stretch and loosen up before they even begin their warm-up, and then they go through at least a forty-five-minute warm-up session that really gets them ready to play from the first hole on. Amateur golfers often go straight from the car to the first tee and can't figure out why their rounds get off to such a bad start.

"The pros all hit a few putts before they go to the practice tee to warm up. I really think they do this for two reasons. First, putting is the most important part of golf—you will cost yourself more strokes with putting woes than anywhere else. Second, you don't want to have a long time pass from the time you warm up until the time you tee off, so the pros practice putting for maybe thirty minutes, then warm up by hitting balls for thirty-five minutes, then pitch, chip, and hit sand shots for ten minutes, then maybe get in another ten minutes of putting before they go to the tee. This keeps the time from the last full swing in warm-ups until the first full shot on the course to a minimum."

BENEFITS OF A PROPER WARM-UP

- Increases blood flow to the muscles
- Increases the core body temperature
- Prepares the neuromuscular system, supporting better coordination
- Promotes flexibility and strength
- Reduces the risk of injury
- Prepares you mentally and boosts confidence

Pre-round Flexibility Conditioning

To effectively prepare the body for golf we utilize dynamic rather than static movements. Each stretch is held for two to five deep breaths, or approximately five to ten seconds. Dynamic stretches "alert" the neuromuscular system for the golf swing more effectively than static stretching does. Dynamic movement raises your core temperature, coordinates movement and breathing (great for rhythm and tempo), and supports mental focus.

Guidelines for Dynamic Stretching

- Breathe in and out through the nose.
- Do not bounce in the stretch.
- Slight discomfort is acceptable, but you should never experience pain while stretching.
- Do not stretch injured or overstretched joints and muscles.
- Flex or engage the opposing muscle. For example, while stretching the hamstrings, engage or flex the quads.
- Stretch before, during, and after your round to develop and maintain optimal muscle balance.

A comprehensive warm-up should target the following areas:

- Core/torso
- Feet, ankles, and calves
- Hips
- Back—including the upper back, shoulders, and chest
- Hamstrings
- Hands and wrists
- Neck

Fitness note: In the following section, exercises denoted with the letter "T" are suggested as a warm-up for traveling golfers. Exercises followed by "OC" are suggested as on-course or practice-tee warm-ups.

LYING WARM-UP SERIES

Pelvic Tilts

With your knees bent and your feet flat on the floor, inhale and bring your lower back into a neutral position. Exhale as you press your lower back toward the floor and tilt the pelvis toward the ceiling. Repeat ten times.

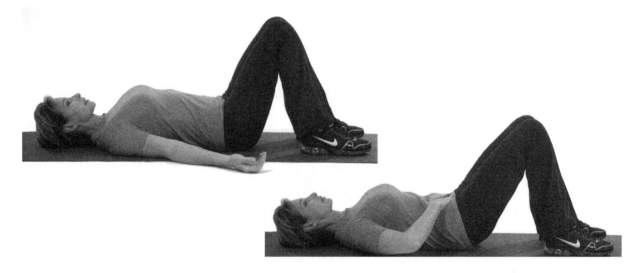

Knees to Chest (T)

Inhale as you bring your arms above your head. Exhale as you pull your right knee to your chest and your head to your knee. Switch sides and repeat ten times.

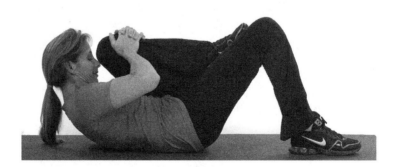

Spinal Rotation with Arms Perpendicular to the Body (T)

Inhale as you bring your legs to the right, keeping your shoulders in contact with the floor. Exhale, initiating the movement from your oblique abdominal muscles, and bring the legs back to the starting position. Switch sides and repeat ten times in each direction. To make this more challenging, lift your legs off the floor, with your knees at a 90-degree angle.

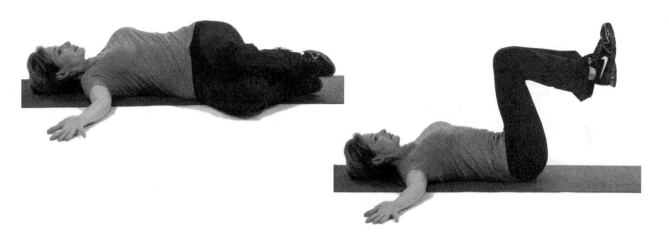

Dynamic Window Washers—Internal/External Hip Stretch

Begin with your feet wider than hip-width apart. Inhale as you bring both knees to the right, then exhale as you return to the starting position. Switch sides and repeat five times in each direction.

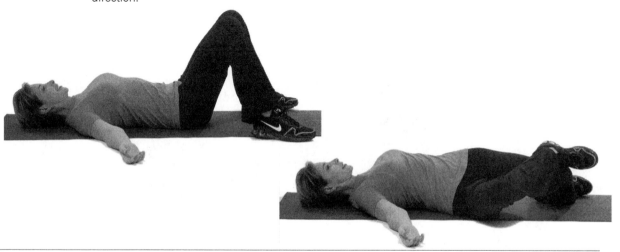

Cat/Cow Spinal Warm-up (T)

Place your hands directly under your shoulders and your knees directly under your hips. Spread your fingers as wide as possible and press your entire hand into the floor. Inhale as you press your spine toward the floor and slightly lift your head, then exhale as you pull your navel toward your spine, engage your glutes, press your spine toward the ceiling, and tuck your chin into your chest. Repeat ten times.

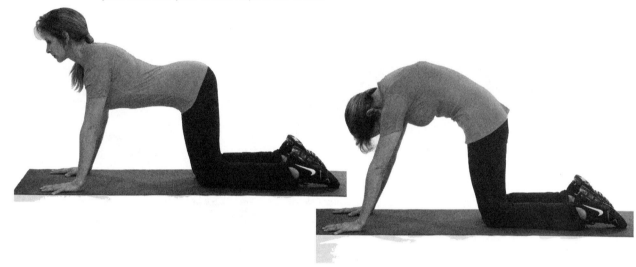

Articulating Bridge Position

Bend your knees until your feet are approximately one foot from your glutes. Inhale as you press your lumbar spine toward the floor and engage the glutes. Exhale as you lift your hips off the floor, one vertebra at a time. Reverse the movement as you lower your glutes back to the floor. Repeat five to ten times.

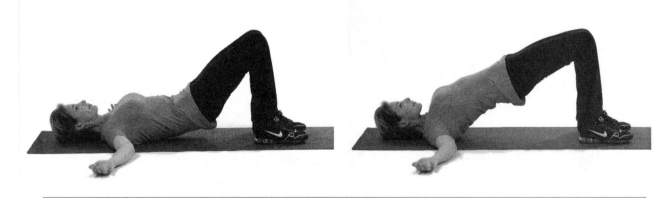

Supine Spinal/Hip Disassociation Stretch (T)

Lie on your side and rest on your right shoulder, then bring your knees to a 90-degree angle. Support your head and neck with a towel. Bring the arms to shoulder height, palms together. Maintain a connection between the knees. Inhale deeply and on your exhale roll the upper body open, bringing the left arm as close to the floor as possible. Measure the distance from your left shoulder to the floor and measure the point at which your back immobility causes your knees to separate. Switch sides and repeat.

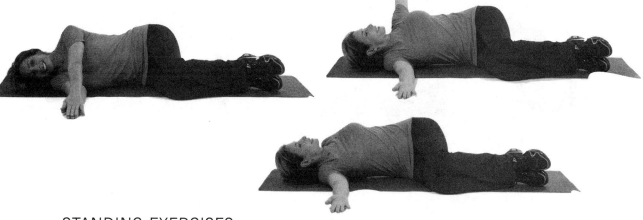

STANDING EXERCISES

Hip and Shoulder Warm-up (T)

Begin in a lunge position, and then extend your arms to shoulder height. Spread your fingers wide and circle your arms clockwise for ten repetitions, counterclockwise for another ten reps. Press the arms forward and backward in small, compact movements ten times.

Keep your arms extended and rotate slowly from your trunk, keeping your hips stable and stationary. When you feel your torso is warmed up, increase the speed of this rotation and repeat for ten more reps. Switch sides.

Hip/Trunk/Lat Extension

Begin in a lunge position and place a golf club in your left hand. Stretch the shoulder, lats, and hip on the right side. Hold for three breaths, repeat three times, and switch sides.

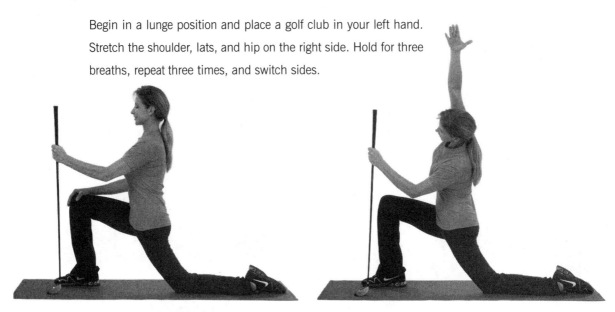

Standing Pelvic Tilts (OC)

Begin in your address position, with your arms crossed over your chest. Make a slight posterior tilt in the hips and pelvis, arch your back (creating an anterior tilt of the hips and pelvis), and return to a neutral spine. Repeat five times in each direction.

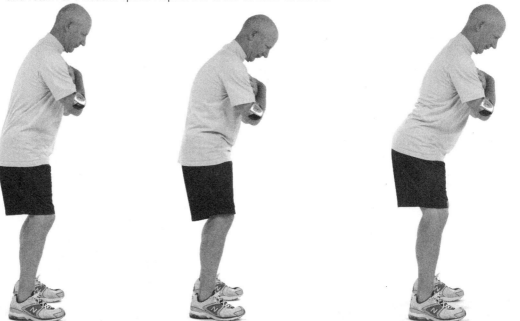

Speed Trunk Rotation (OC)

While standing in your address position, bring your palms together. Inhale as you rotate from the core and bring your right arm back. Exhale as you "clap" your hands together. Repeat ten times in each direction.

Continuing in your address position, extend the arms to shoulder height and rotate from the core. Repeat ten more times.

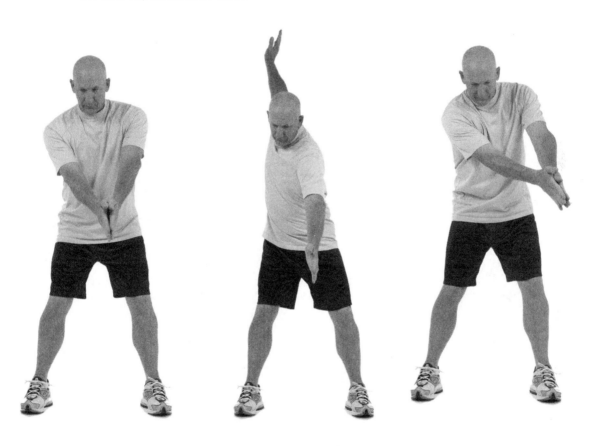

Standing Glute/Hip Stretch (OC)

Begin by placing your hands on a chair or a golf club to help you maintain your balance. Place your right ankle on the outside of your left knee. Inhale as you bend your left knee, sitting back as if you were sitting on a chair. Bring your chest toward your shin, rolling your shoulder blades together. Hold for three breaths and repeat five times. Switch sides.

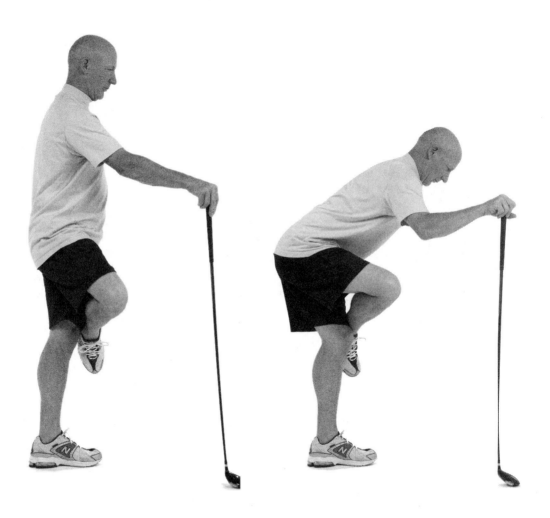

Shoulder Stretch with Club Behind Back (OC)

Place a club or a towel in your right hand, with the palm facing the ceiling. Bring your right arm over your head and your right palm behind your back. Bring your left arm behind your back and clasp the club or towel. Inhale as you gently pull on the club or towel with your left arm, then exhale and release. Repeat five times and switch arms.

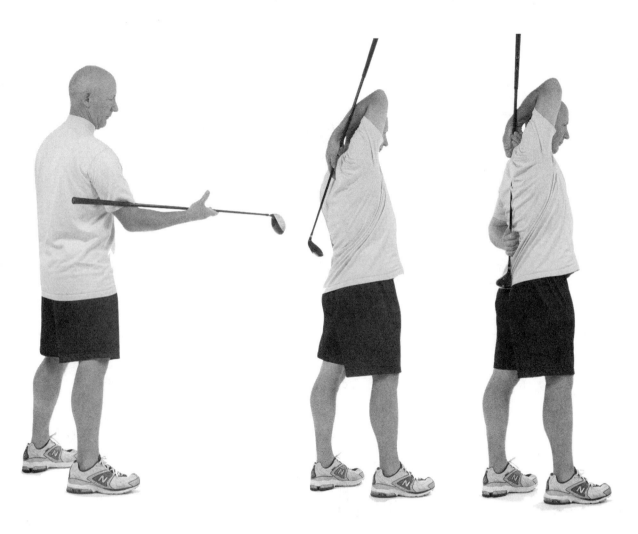

Neck Stretch, Pressing Opposite Hand Toward the Floor

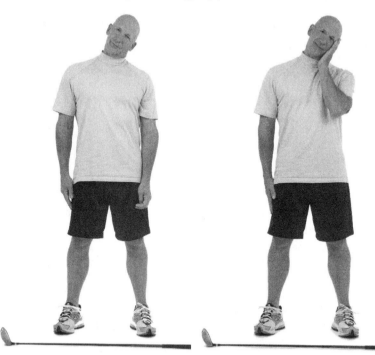

Bring your left ear toward your left shoulder as you continue to face forward. Inhale as you press your right arm toward the floor using your left hand to gently support your head. Hold for five breaths and use your left hand to gently return your head and neck to neutral. Switch sides.

Standing Rhomboid/Upper Back/Neck Stretch (OC)

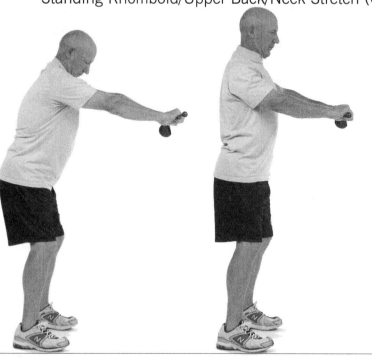

Bring a club to shoulder height, bend your knees, and tuck your pelvis under. Inhale as you press your arms away from you, tucking your chin into your chest. Exhale, lift your head, and squeeze your shoulder blades together. Repeat five times.

SECTION TWO

FIXING THE GOLF SWING'S MOST TROUBLESOME FLAWS

CHAPTER SIX
THE "S" POSTURE
SWING FLAW

When I want a long ball, I spin my hips faster.

— JACK NICKLAUS

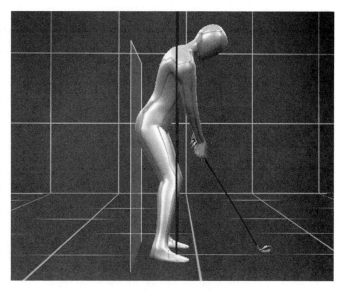

THE "S" POSTURE refers to the shape of the lumbar spine, specifically a curve or excessive arch in the lumbar spine that resembles the letter "s." This condition often causes pain in the lumbar spine, weakens the abdominals, and compromises lumbar and hip mobility. The "S" curve creates inefficient lower-body power because the hips cannot transfer energy to the trunk. Fitness professionals also refer to this condition as an excessive arch in the lumbar spine, which creates an anterior tilt of the pelvis. Without the ability to create a posterior tilt (the opposite of an anterior tilt) in the pelvis, the transition of power through impact and glute activation is compromised. Through 3D motion analysis we know that most Tour players have their hips leaning back at impact, which helps them generate power from the lower body. If you can't tuck the pelvis under, due to an excessive "S" posture, or create a posterior tilt you will prevent your body from generating maximum power.

HANK'S PERSPECTIVE

There are many important angles in the golf swing, and the swing plane is probably the most important one. Every golfer has a correct swing plane that they need to swing the club on, and this plane is established by the angle of the clubshaft at address. The second most important angle in the golf swing is the angle of your body, i.e., your posture. Ideally, you'll set up with one posture and address and maintain it throughout the swing. The angle of your clubshaft, your swing plane, and your posture determine the amount of ground that you will hit when you swing the golf club, and everything must be matched properly in order to have a consistent swing that hits the correct amount of ground. The best way for this to happen is for a golfer to swing the club on his or her correct swing plane while maintaining the correct posture that was established at address.

The hips are obviously very important to your swing. The hips are part of your core, and your core really anchors your swing. If you don't position the hips properly at address and keep them there as you rotate, it will be impossible to have a powerful and repeating swing. The hips need to resist in the backswing to build coil and lead in the downswing to provide power and timing.

FITNESS SOLUTIONS

These exercises will help you alleviate the "S" curve in your spine and help you develop more mobility in the hips, thus keeping your posture intact throughout your swing.

Strength and mobility in the glutes are fundamental to reducing the "S" curve in your spine.

Pelvic Tilts

Begin on your back with your knees bent and your feet flat on the floor. Inhale as you bring the lower spine into a neutral position. Exhale as you press your lower back toward the floor and tilt your pelvis toward the ceiling. Repeat ten times.

Articulating Bridge Position

Bend your knees until your feet are approximately one foot from your glutes. Inhale as you press your lumbar spine toward the floor and engage the glutes. Exhale as you lift your hips off the floor, one vertebra at a time. Reverse the movement as you lower your glutes back to the floor. Repeat five to ten times.

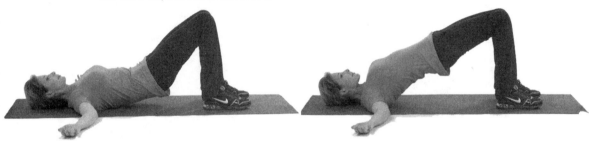

Cat/Cow Spinal Warm-up

Place your hands directly under your shoulders and your knees directly under your hips. Spread your fingers as wide as possible, pressing your entire hand into the floor. Inhale as you press your spine toward the floor and slightly lift your head, then exhale as you pull your navel toward your spine, engage your glutes, press your spine toward the ceiling, and tuck your chin into your chest. Repeat ten times.

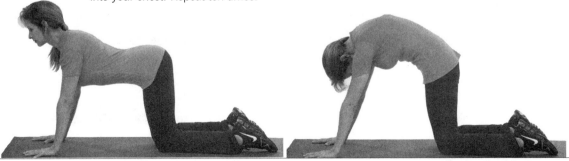

Internal/External Hip Stretch

Begin with your feet wider than hip-width apart. Inhale as you bring both knees to the right, then exhale as you return to the starting position. Switch sides and repeat five times in each direction.

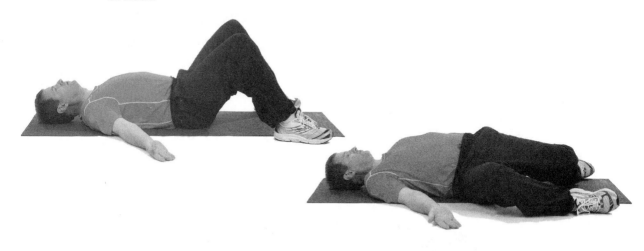

Dynamic Supine External Hip Stretch with Ball

Place your right foot on a stability ball and your left ankle outside your right knee. On your exhalation roll the ball toward you, focusing on the stretch in the left hip. Repeat five to ten times and switch sides.

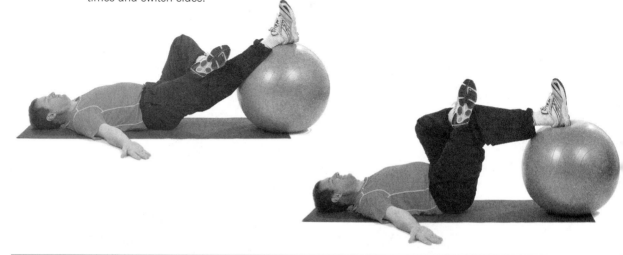

Glute Strengthener: Bridge Exercise with Leg Lifts

Lie on the ground, place your feet hip-width apart, bend your knees, and lift your hips up off the floor. To make this more challenging, you can extend one of your legs at the same level as your opposite knee and hold for a count of ten. To make it even harder, you can move that extended leg up and down. Switch sides so both glutes are equally strengthened.

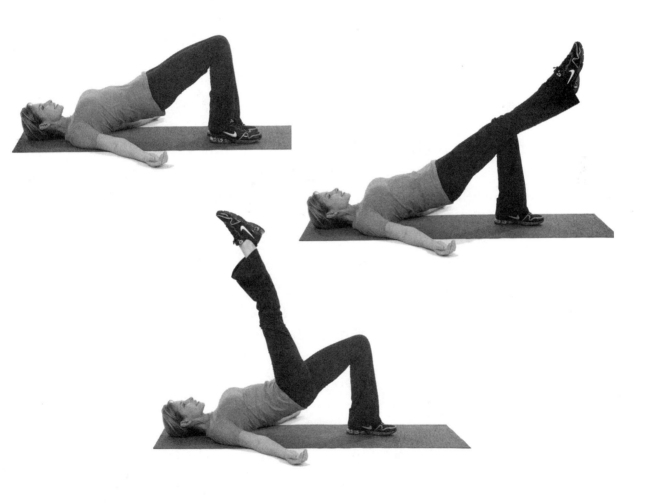

Standing Quad Stretch

Place your right foot on the seat of a chair, with a club in your left hand to help you maintain your balance. The hips should face forward and the knees should be aligned. Engage your right glute and press your right hip forward. Hold for five breaths, relax, and repeat three times. Switch sides.

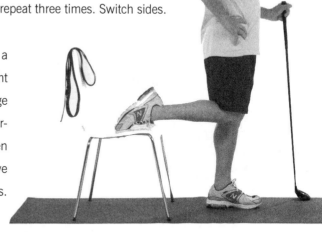

To make it more challenging, place a strap around your left foot and your right hand on the back of the chair. Engage the left glute and press your left hip forward. Gently create resistance between the strap and your foot. Hold for five breaths, relax, and repeat three times. Switch sides.

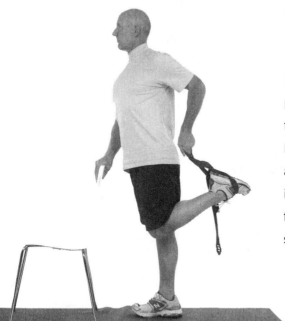

For maximum challenge, place the top of your left foot into your left palm. Press the left hip forward and gently press your foot into your hand. Hold for five breaths and switch sides. Repeat two times.

CHAPTER SEVEN
"C" POSTURE— SWING FLAW

Swinging the club is like swinging an axe. You do not hit with it; you accelerate with it.

—PETER THOMSON

"C POSTURE" IS ONE of the most common physical restrictions I see in my golfers. The name comes from the rounded back and slumped shoulders that make the upper back resemble the letter "c." It's often accompanied by the excessive forward lean of the head. These two issues restrict efficient spinal mobility. In my opinion the "C" posture is primarily a by-product of our sedentary lifestyle. Sitting too much, the aging process, and an imbalanced fitness program (heavy upper-body lifting without flexibility conditioning) create an imbalance in the chest and upper-back musculature.

The solution to the "C" posture is to build flexibility in the front of the body and strength in the back of the body. Mobility in the spine is essential, specifically the ability to generate extension. Without proper balance in the upper spine you will find it difficult to rotate, which prevents you from separating your shoulders from your hips, which is the root of power in the swing. Note: Improperly fitted clubs may cause a "C" posture at address.

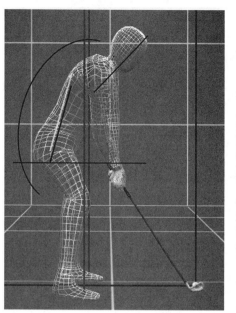 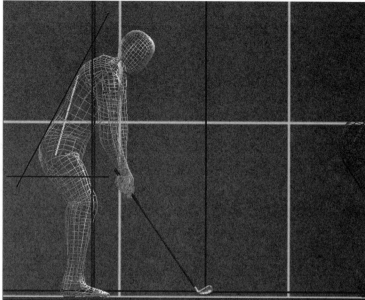

HANK'S PERSPECTIVE

In the proper address position your shoulders should be pulled back, not slouched forward. Setting up with your shoulders forward is easy to do because the ball is out in front of us at address, but ideally your shoulders should be pulled back at address and remain that way throughout the swing. This helps to establish and define a posture that is not only correct but also repeatable. Another benefit of having your shoulders pulled back is that is allows your upper arms to stay connected to your chest. This connection is an important part of getting your arms and body to work together in the golf swing. A connected swing is a key to having a correct swing, and being connected starts with a correct posture at address.

As far as your head position is concerned, it's important that your head stay centered as your body rotates around the central axis of your swing. One of the most important things that I look for in a golf swing is the eyes remaining parallel to the target line and level to the ground throughout the swing. Eye level is particularly important, because one contributing factor to good balance is the ability to keep your eyes level to the horizon—if your eyes tilt a lot during the swing, your balance will be affected in a negative way.

FITNESS SOLUTIONS

Supine Chest Stretch on the Ball

Roll a stability ball behind your upper spine, supporting your head. Lift your hips and engage your glutes until your lower body is parallel to the floor. Your arms should be at a 90-degree angle, pressing away from the ceiling and focusing on the stretch in the chest and mid-back. Hold for ten deep breaths.

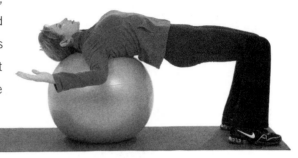

Supine Thoracic Spine Mobility Stretch

Begin with your legs resting on the seat of a chair and your hands clasped above your chest. Press your navel toward your spine and extend your arms over your head. Hold for five breaths and repeat three times.

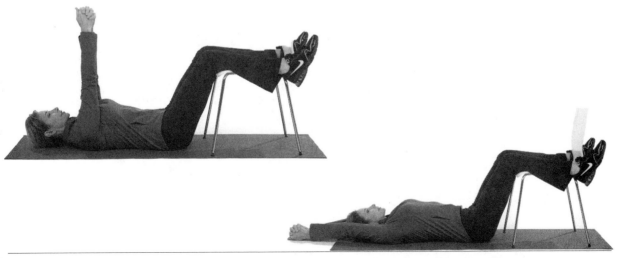

Pec/Upper-Back Extension

Stand with your hands clasped behind your head. Inhale as you squeeze your elbows together, exhale, and then press your elbows back. Repeat five times.

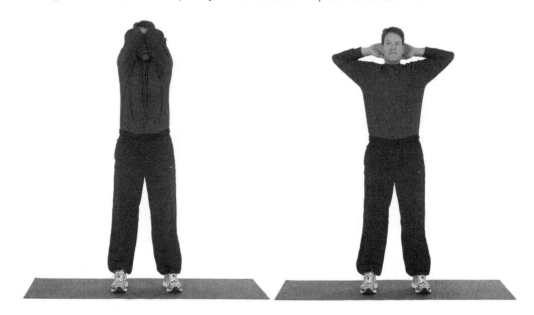

Neck Stretch, Pressing Opposite Hand Toward The Floor

Bring your left ear toward your left shoulder as you continue to face forward. Inhale as you press your right arm toward the floor using your left hand to gently support your head. Hold for five breaths and use your left hand to gently return your head and neck to neutral. Switch sides.

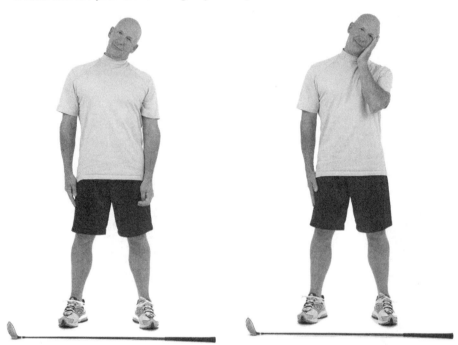

Arm Glides

Begin on your back with your knees bent, your arms perpendicular to your body, and your elbows bent at a 90-degree angle. Exhale and glide your arms across the floor and over your head. Repeat five to ten times.

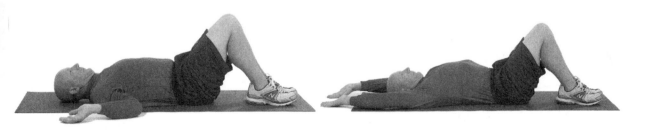

Standing Rhomboid/Mid-back Muscles Stretching and Strengthening Exercise with Golf Club

Place a club in your hands, which should be shoulder-width apart. Inhale as you press your arms forward, tucking your chin into your chest and keeping your shoulders down. Exhale as you squeeze your shoulder blades together. Repeat five to ten times.

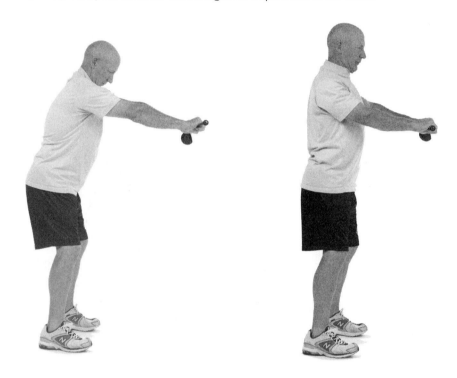

Posture Exercise with Golf Club

Place a club along your spine. Bend forward, hinging at the hips, with your knees slightly bent. Maintain a connection between your entire spine and the club.

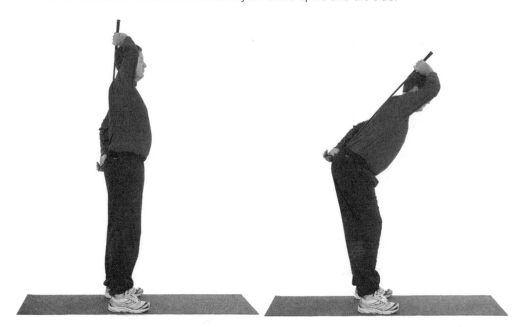

Lat Stretch

Begin by sitting on your heels, with your knees on the ground. (If you have discomfort in your knees, place a rolled up towel behind them.) Stretch your arms forward, shoulder-width apart, until they touch the floor in front of you, then go up onto your fingertips. Stretch your arms to the right, bringing your right arm perpendicular to your right hip. Maintain the connection between your left glute and your left heel. Hold for five breaths and switch sides.

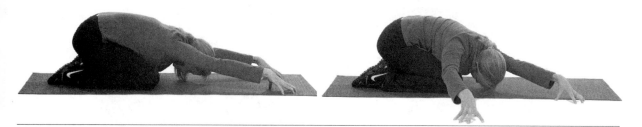

Modified Cobra

Begin with your hands placed next to your chest, your legs together, and the tops of your feet on the floor. Inhale as you squeeze your legs together, activating the glutes. Exhale as you lift your chest off the floor. Repeat dynamically five times. Hold for five more breaths, focusing on activating the rhomboid muscles. Keep your shoulders moving down, away from your ears.

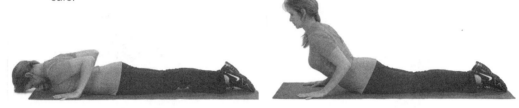

Twisting Table

Begin on all fours, with your right hand placed on your head and your right elbow pulled up behind your head. Inhale and twist from the thoracic spine toward the ceiling. Exhale and tuck your right shoulder under your left shoulder. Repeat five times and hold the right arm tucked under your left shoulder for five more breaths.

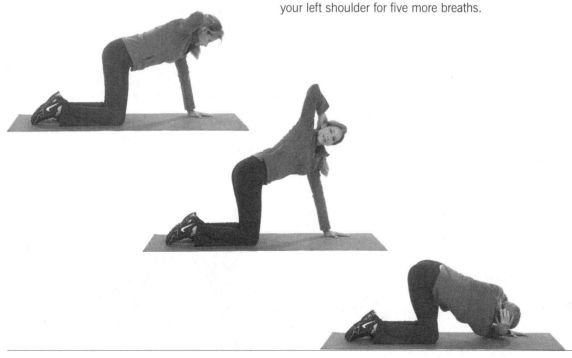

Rear Delt Exercises Prone on the Ball

Place a stability ball under your hips. Squeeze your legs together to stabilize the lower body. Lift your chest off the ball, thumbs facing the ceiling, arms extended slightly wider than shoulder-width apart. Lift the arms five to ten times. Rest for one minute.

Bring your arms perpendicular to your shoulders.

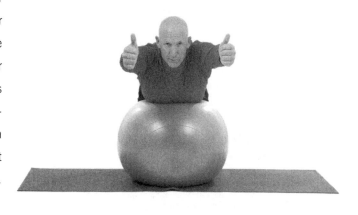

Lift the arms five to ten times. Rest for one minute. Bring the arms behind your body to a 45-degree angle, thumbs facing the ceiling.

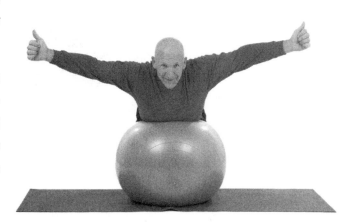

Lift the arms five to ten times. Rest for one minute.

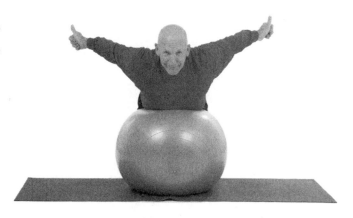

Static Shoulder/Hip Disassociation Stretch

Begin by lying on your right side with your arms extended and your palms together. Place your legs at a 90-degree angle to your body, knees together. Roll the left shoulder toward the floor. If your shoulder does not contact the floor, place a towel under your shoulder. Relax in this position for three minutes, focusing on your breathing. Release tension in your body with every exhalation.

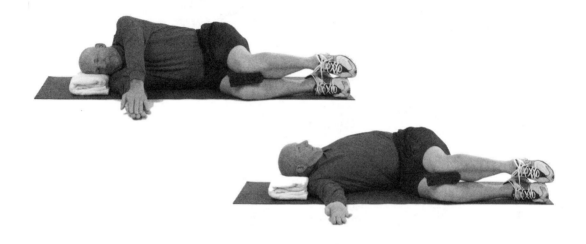

CHAPTER EIGHT
LOSS OF POSTURE/ LIFTING UP

The most important shot in golf is the next one.

—BEN HOGAN

LOSS OF POSTURE" or "lifting up" is an inability to maintain a consistent spine angle throughout the swing; it primarily involves a change in the spine angle from the address position through the full swing. The proper golf swing occurs when the torso rotates around the axis of the spine. Many golfers believe a loss of posture or lifting up is primarily due to poor mechanics, but the physical causes of this fault are lack of core mobility and strength, as well as instability in the lower body. My experience with many golfers is that when we see hip mobility issues such as an elevated hip or lack of mobility, the dysfunction directly affects shoulder mobility. Specifically, tension in the hip flexors makes the ability to rotate around the right side difficult, and the core compensates by lifting up out of the address position. Additionally, compromised torso mobility makes it difficult to generate the necessary separation between the upper and lower body.

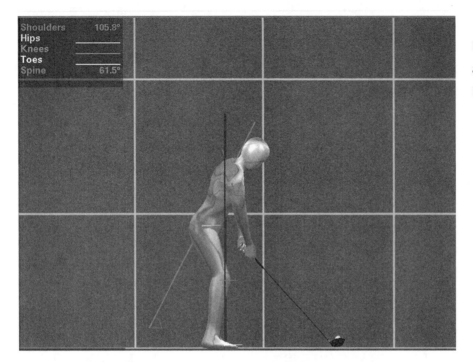

Note the spine angle at address is 61.5 degrees.

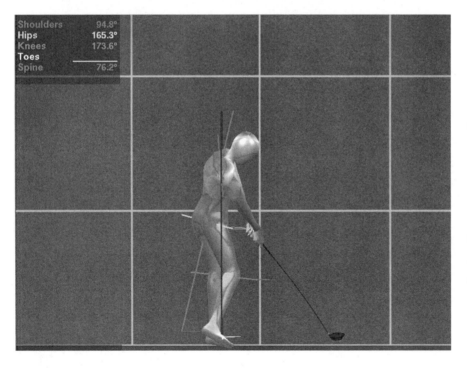

Note the change in the golfer's spine angle. He has lifted up and has lost his original spine angle. Motion analysis shows a 14.7-degree variation from address to impact.

HANK'S PERSPECTIVE

One of the most common mistakes that golfers make is that they come out of their posture during the swing, particularly as the club is coming into impact. There can be many reasons why you come out of your posture—for example, swinging the club on too steep of a swing plane can force you to come out of your posture so that you don't hit too much ground. But it's usually a lack of core strength that makes golfers lose their posture, and this results in thin shots or a topped golf ball.

FITNESS SOLUTIONS

Lat Stretch to Lat Strengthener

Begin by sitting on your heels, with your knees on the ground. (If you have discomfort in your knees, place a rolled-up towel behind them.) Stretch your arms forward, wider than shoulder-width apart, until they touch the floor in front of you, palms facing inward.

Lift your right arm off the floor. Hold for five breaths and switch sides. Repeat three times.

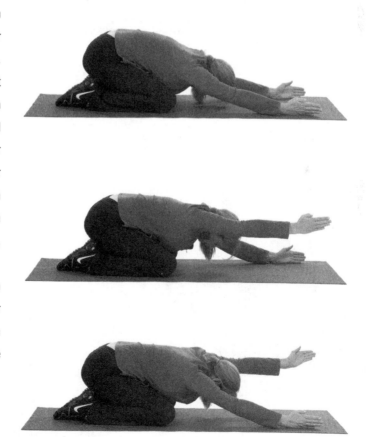

The Turn

Begin on your back with your knees bent, your feet on the floor, and a stability ball in your hands. Inhale as you roll your arms to the left and your legs to the right. Exhale as you return to the starting position. Make sure you initiate the movement from your oblique abdominals. Switch sides and repeat five times.

To make it more challenging, you can lift your legs off the floor.

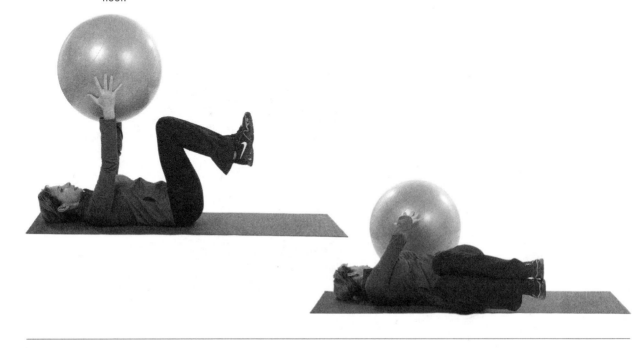

4 x 4 Hip Stretch

Place your left ankle over your right knee. Press your left knee away from your body. Hold for five breaths and switch sides. To make it more challenging, you can place a strap around your right hamstring and lift your right leg off the floor.

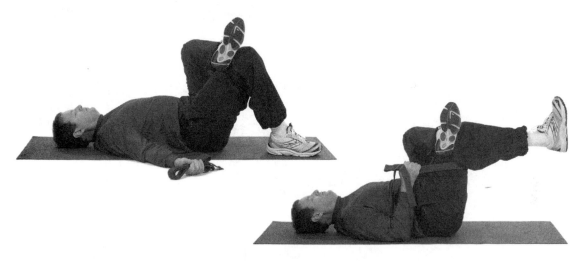

Groin Stretch

Sit with your back against a wall and the soles of your feet together. Bring your feet as close as possible to your groin and hold for three minutes.

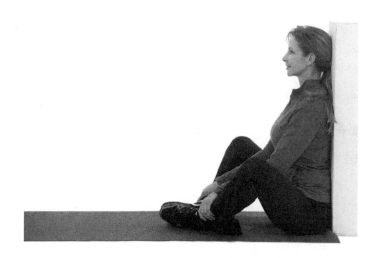

Core-Stabilizing Series

Begin on your back, with your knees bent and a towel between your hands. Press your navel to your spine while your lower back and rib cage remain connected to the floor. Lift your right foot one inch off the floor. Slowly switch sides and repeat five times.

To make this more challenging, raise your left leg off the floor with your knee at a 90-degree angle as you lift your right leg off the floor. On your exhalation switch sides. Repeat five times.

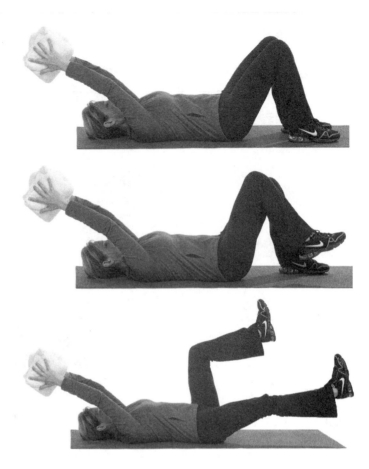

Pilates Roll-downs

Squeeze a stability ball between your hands. Inhale as you articulate your spine down to the floor. When your bottom rib touches the floor, exhale and roll back to the starting position. Repeat ten to twenty times.

To make this more challenging, when you get to the point at which you abs are involved, rotate from your core and bring the ball to the right and left.

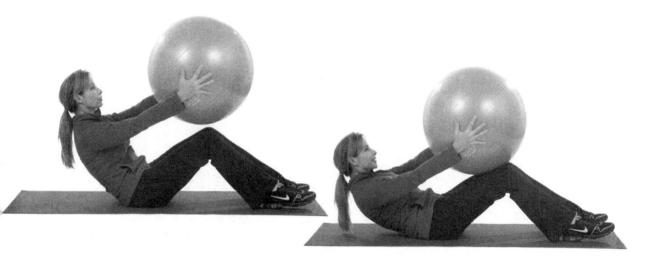

Exhale and return to the starting position. Switch sides. Once you have mastered the movement, speed up the action to a more explosive movement.

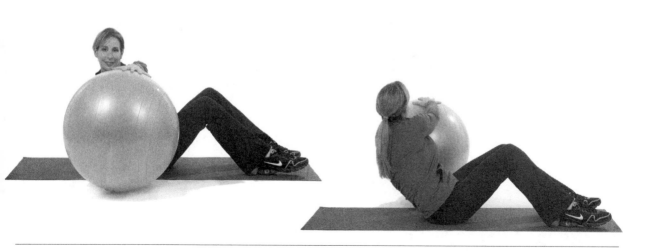

Core Crunch with Ball

Begin by lying on your back with your knees bent and your hands clasped behind your head to support your neck. Place a ball or towel between your knees. On your exhale, lift your chest off the floor. Repeat until you feel muscle fatigue. To make it more challenging, you can squeeze the upper and lower body together.

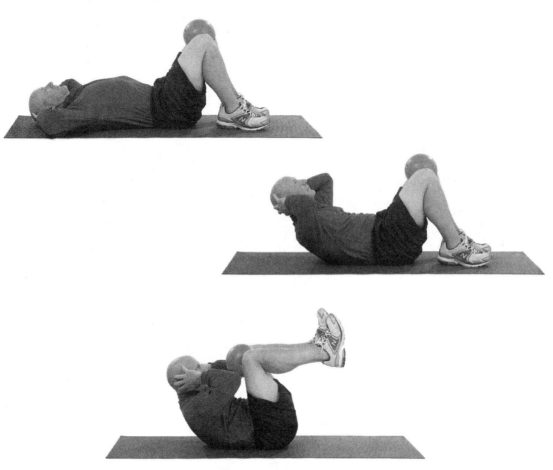

Extended Table

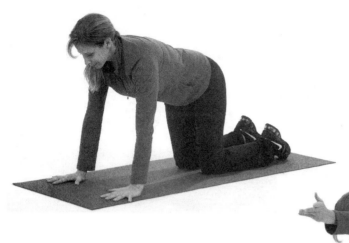

Begin on all fours and stabilize your core by pulling your navel toward your spine. Extend your left arm and right leg. Lift the leg and arm as high as possible without arching your back. Hold for thirty seconds and switch sides. Repeat three times.

Modified Cobra

Begin with your hands placed next to your chest, your legs together, and the tops of your feet on the floor. Inhale as you squeeze your legs together, activating the glutes. Exhale as you lift your chest off the floor. Repeat dynamically five times. Hold for five more breaths, focusing on activating the mid-back muscles. Keep your shoulders moving down, away from your ears.

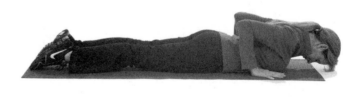

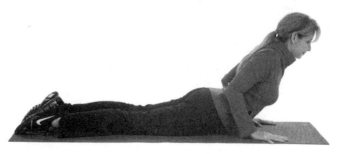

Plank

Place your hands directly under your shoulders, spread your fingers wide, and press your palms into the floor. Lift your knees off the floor and 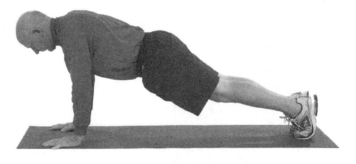 bring the body parallel to the floor, into a plank position. Maintain this position without letting your back sag for thirty seconds to one minute. Repeat three times.

Dynamic Shoulder/Hip Disassociation Stretch

Begin by lying on your right side, with your arms extended and your palms together. Place your legs at a 90-degree angle to your body, knees together. Roll the left shoulder toward the floor. If your shoulder does not contact the floor, place a towel under your shoulder. Relax in

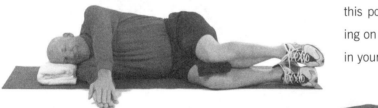

this position for three minutes, focusing on your breathing. Release tension in your body with every exhalation.

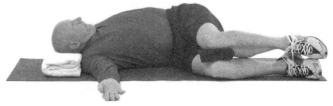

Passive Hip Release with One Leg on the Chair

Place your left leg on the seat of a chair and your right leg on the floor. Hold for three to five minutes and switch sides.

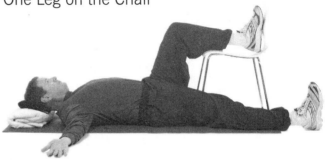

CHAPTER NINE
SWAY SWING FLAW

When a player steps to hit the ball he should be thinking of nothing
else in the world than hitting the ball. By that time he must have put
out of his mind any thought of whether he is taking the club back right,
whether he is hurrying the backswing, whether his grip is correct . . .
or any of the other things that may enter into the correct making of
the stroke.

—GENE SARAZEN

A POWERFUL GOLF SWING is one in which the spine coils efficiently. During
the takeaway, approximately 75 percent of your weight transfers to the
right leg. The trunk, arms, and pelvis begin to rotate, which starts the
"coiling" of the spine. At this point we begin to experience the relationship between
the spine and the right hip.

As the golfer moves into the top of the backswing, the upper body begins to
twist vertically while the lower body twists horizontally. The right hip and lower
body are activated. In Tour players we see the lower body activation occur before
the player reaches the full backswing. This coiling in different directions generates
power, but it can also cause injury.

Sway occurs when the lower body moves laterally to the right (in a right-handed golfer) instead of coiling around the axis of the spine. A golfer's leg will often lock and the weight will shift to the outside of the right foot. It is common to see an exaggerated sway causing another swing flaw, the reverse pivot. A sway shifts all of the weight to the right side, making it challenging to transition to the proper downswing. Physically, a sway is caused by the inability to internally rotate the hips due to a lack of flexibility, as well as to a lack of strength in the glutes. Poor strength inhibits control of the hips and depletes power and distance. To resolve sway it is critical to have mobility and strength in the hips and glutes and range of motion in the trunk.

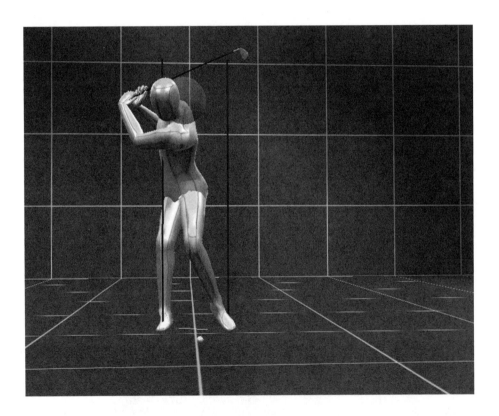

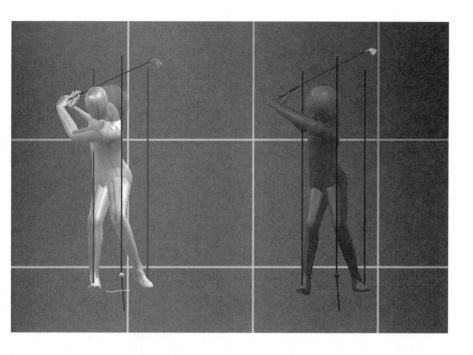

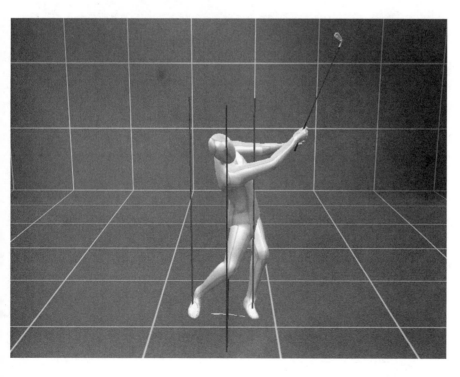

This image
demonstrates
slide, sway in the
finish position.

PHYSICAL FACTORS AFFECTING SWAY

Hip adduction (inner thigh) and abduction (outer thigh) mobility

Glute and lower-body strength

Trunk mobility

Lack of shoulder turn

Lack of strength in the glutes

HANK'S PERSPECTIVE

When a golfer sways they are not turning around the central axis of their body. Ideally you would rotate around this axis and make a tight and compact turn. Your shoulders should turn on top of your hips and your head should stay pretty much stationary. Golfers often sway instead of turning because their flexibility inhibits their ability to turn. A sway is never as powerful or as repeating as a coiled turn. A coiled turn is one in which the lower body resists and the upper body turns. Imagine a top that is spinning fast—it spins in a tight area, but as it slows down it starts to sway back and forth. It's the same for a golfer who sways: They lose potential speed.

FITNESS SOLUTIONS

Internal/External Hip Stretch

Begin with your feet wider than hip-width apart. Inhale as you bring both knees to the right, then exhale as you return to the starting position. Switch sides and repeat five times in each direction.

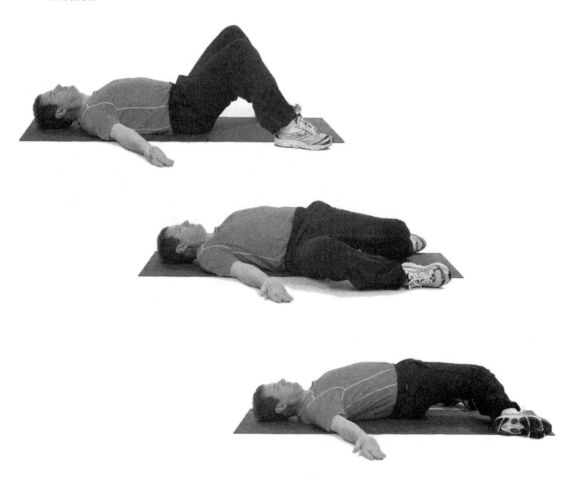

Articulating Bridge Position

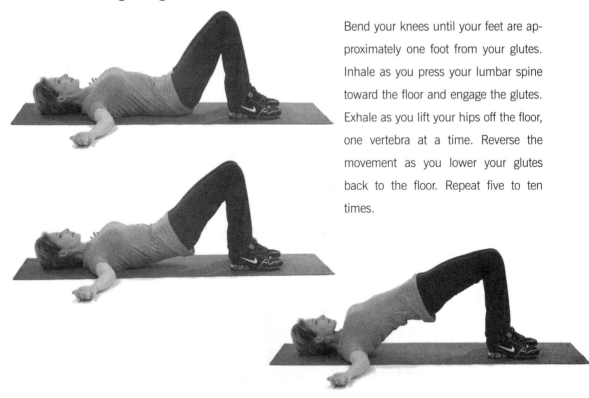

Bend your knees until your feet are approximately one foot from your glutes. Inhale as you press your lumbar spine toward the floor and engage the glutes. Exhale as you lift your hips off the floor, one vertebra at a time. Reverse the movement as you lower your glutes back to the floor. Repeat five to ten times.

4 x 4 Hip Stretch

Place your left ankle over your right knee. Press your left knee away from your body. Hold for five breaths and switch sides. To make it more challenging, you can place a strap around your right hamstring and lift your right leg off the floor.

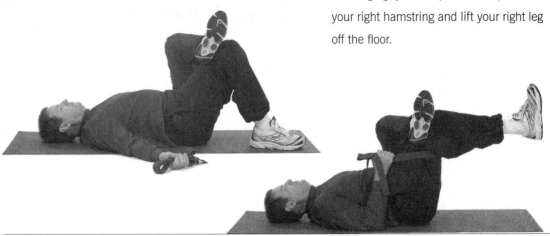

Spinal/Hip/Hamstring Series with Strap

Place a strap or belt around your right foot and extend your left leg. Flex both feet and activate both quads. Press your left hip toward the floor and extend your left arm perpendicular to your body. Hold for five breaths. Extend your right leg to the right, maintaining connection between your left glute and the floor. Hold for five breaths.

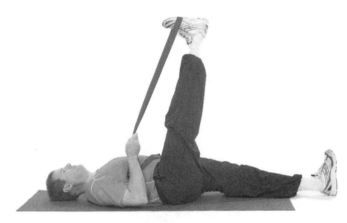

Place the strap in your left hand, extend your right arm perpendicular to your body, and bring your right leg and hip to the left, focusing on the spinal rotation. Hold for five breaths and switch sides.

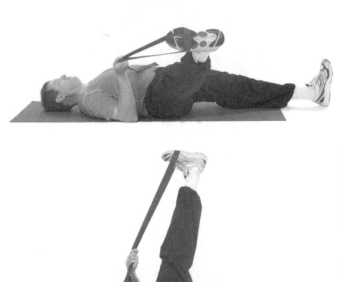

Dynamic Shoulder/Hip Disassociation Stretch

Begin by lying on your right side, with your arms extended and your palms together. Place your legs at a 90-degree angle to your body, knees together. Roll the left shoulder toward the floor. If your shoulder does not contact the floor, place a towel under your shoulder. Inhale, bringing the palms back together. Repeat five times and switch sides.

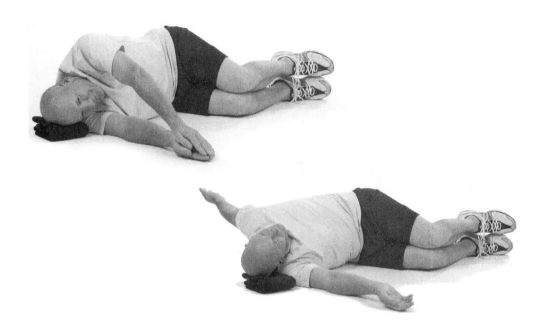

Hip Stability/Torso Mobility Exercise

Place your left knee on the floor, with your right leg at a 90-degree angle. Place a club across your chest and stabilize the hips. Rotate your torso to the right and the left. Move with control, focusing on the range of motion in the trunk and stabilizing the hips. Repeat five times in each direction and switch sides.

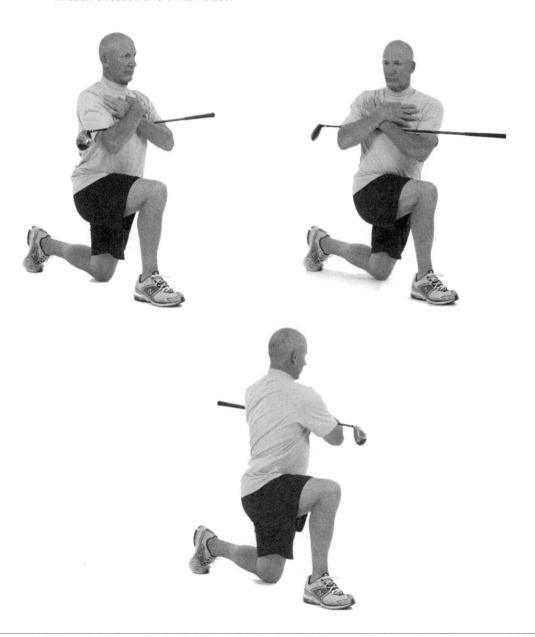

Squats

Stand tall with a chair or stability ball placed about a foot behind you, engaging N.T.R. (navel in, tailbone down, rib cage lifts). Inhale as you "sit" down until your glutes touch the ball or the seat of the chair. Make sure you maintain an upright posture. Exhale and return to the starting position. Repeat ten times.

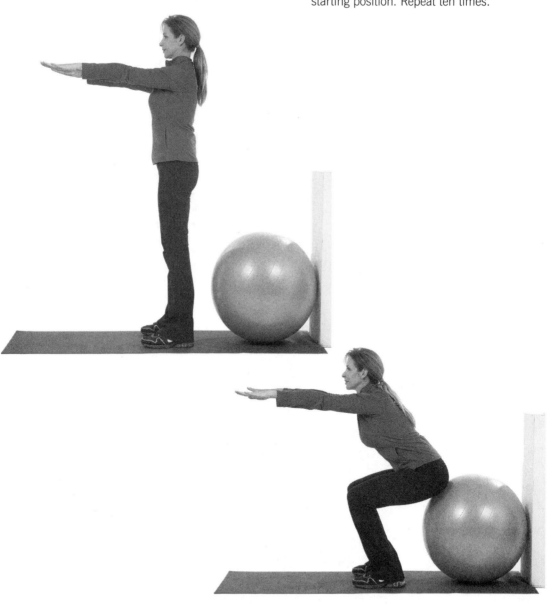

Three-Point Dog Leg

Begin on all fours. Lift your right leg, with your knee at a 90-degree angle. Focus on activating the glute and stabilizing the core. Do not arch the back. Bring your right knee to the outside of your left knee. Return to the starting position and repeat ten times. Switch sides.

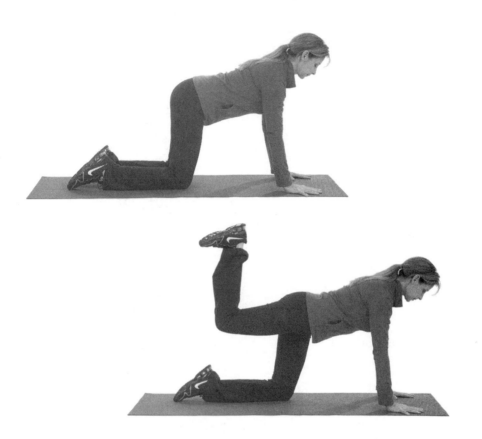

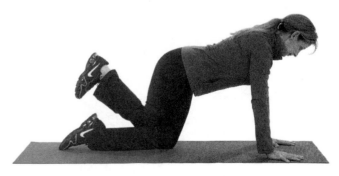

Dynamic Single-Leg Dead Lifts

Place a club at shoulder height and lift your arms over your head. Step your left foot forward and begin to bring your body toward the floor. Move your upper body and lower body as if they are one piece. It is acceptable if the right leg comes a foot or so off the floor. Lift back up and tap the right foot to the floor. Repeat the exercise ten times and switch sides.

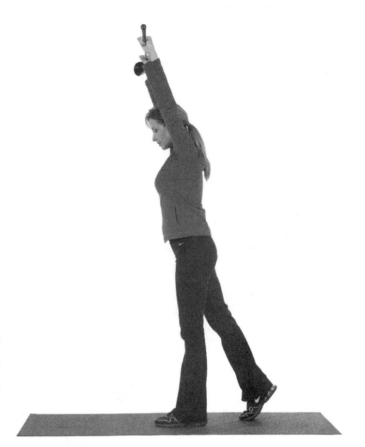

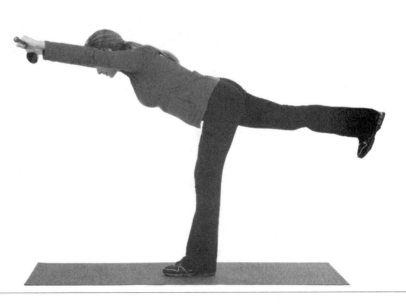

Power Rotation with Club

Place the club at shoulder height. Lunge the left leg to a 90-degree angle and rotate the upper body to the left. Switch sides and repeat five times in each direction.

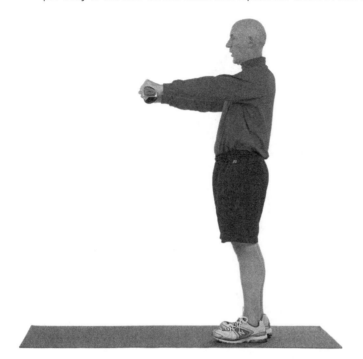

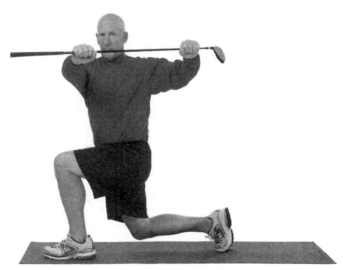

Passive Hip Release with One Leg on the Chair

Place your left leg on the seat of a chair and extend your right leg to the floor. Hold for three to five minutes and switch sides.

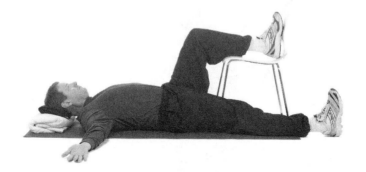

CHAPTER TEN
REVERSE PIVOT—
SWING FLAW

Most golfers prepare for disaster. A good golfer prepares for success.

—Bob Toski

I F YOUR UPPER body bends away from the ball during the downswing, you have a swing fault called a reverse pivot. This causes an interruption in the kinetic link of the swing and creates power loss because the lower body cannot effectively initiate the downswing. If the upper body initiates the downswing, you will hit inconsistent shots and tremendous strain will be placed on the lumbar spine.

This issue is primarily caused by a lack of mobility in the torso. It is important to separate the shoulders and lats from the hips and to fully rotate the spine without excessive side-to-side bending. You also have to use your hips to help you generate rotation. If your hips aren't flexible, this may contribute to a reverse pivot as well.

Core conditioning will stabilize the torso and help you maintain a forward flex of the spine through the entire swing, especially at the top of the backswing, where it is the most important.

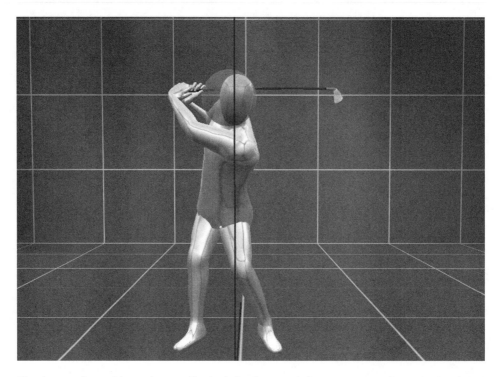

The image shows hip and torso tilts both back toward the target as well as starting head position indicated by circle.

PHYSICAL FIXES

Increase range of motion in the lats and trunk

Hip mobility

Core stability and strength

Glute strength

HANK'S PERSPECTIVE

The reverse pivot is probably the worst mistake that golfers make. You want a little bit of sway in your swing, but a reverse pivot is the complete opposite: It's when the upper body turns toward the target in the backswing as the lower body moves behind the ball. During the backswing you should feel your shoulders turn behind the ball while the lower body stays centered. A reverse pivot is more common with women, because their lower center of gravity makes their hips move back in the backswing, which causes their shoulders to turn toward the target instead of away from it. A reverse pivot in the backswing can also be caused by keeping your head down too much at address, which make your shoulders tilt rather than turn.

FITNESS SOLUTIONS

Supine Shoulder Mobility/Lumbar Stretch

Lie on your back and place your right foot on your left knee and your left hand on your right knee, then rotate your body to the left and bring your right arm to shoulder height. Hold for five deep breaths and switch sides. To make this more challenging, reach your arm over your head.

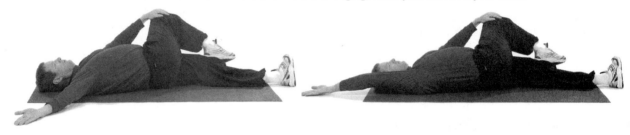

Lat Reach and Roll

Place your hands on a stability ball and activate your core. For more hip stability you can place a towel between your thighs. Stretch your body toward the floor, focusing on the stretch in the lats and shoulders. Hold for one breath in each direction. Repeat five times.

Inhale and roll your upper body to the left, maintaining hip stability. Exhale as you come back to center. Switch sides and repeat five times.

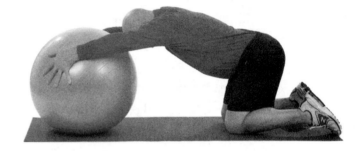

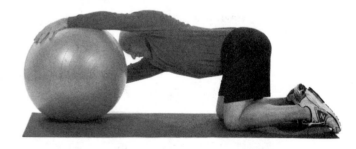

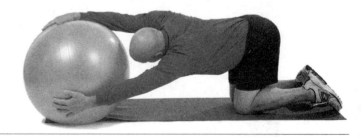

Modified Cobra

Begin with your hands placed next to your chest, your legs together, and the tops of your feet on the floor. Inhale as you squeeze your legs together, activating the glutes. Exhale as you lift your chest off the floor. Repeat dynamically five times. Hold for five more breaths, focusing on activating the rhomboid muscles. Keep your shoulders moving down, away from your ears.

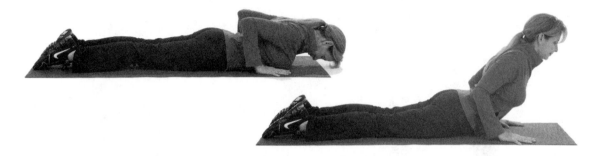

Core-Stabilizing Series

Begin on your back, with your knees bent and a towel between your hands. Press your navel to your spine while your lower back and rib cage remain connected to the floor. Lift your right foot one inch off the floor. Slowly switch sides and repeat five times.

To make this more challenging, raise your left leg off the floor with your knee at a 90-degree angle as you lift your right leg off the floor. On your exhalation, switch sides. Repeat five times.

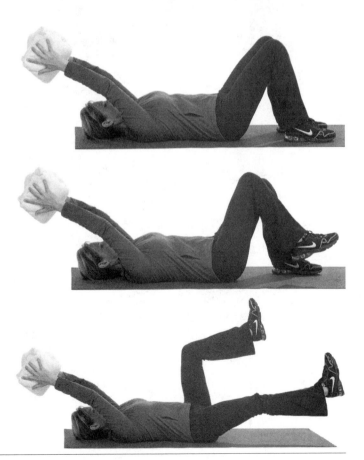

Revolving Shoulder Twist from Lunge

Bring your left knee forward to a lunge position until it's at a 90-degree angle. Bring your right hand to your left knee. Activate N.T.R. (navel in, tailbone down, rib cage lifts) and revolve from the base of your spine. Hold for five breaths and switch sides.

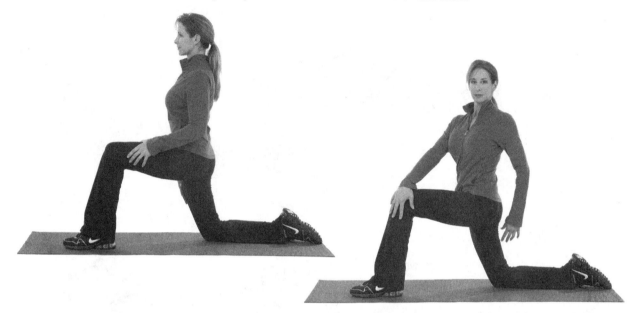

To make it more challenging, put your right elbow on your left knee, your right hand into a fist, and your left hand on top of your right. Twist from the base of your spine, lifting your right shoulder away from your ear. Hold for five breaths and switch sides.

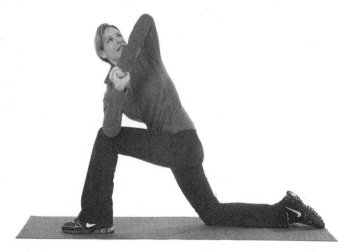

Hip/Trunk/Lat Extension with Club

Lunge your right foot forward with a club in your left hand. Activate N.T.R. and extend your right arm to the ceiling. Exhale as you stretch your right arm over to the left side. Focus on stretching from your right hip, lats, and shoulders. Hold for five deep breaths and switch sides.

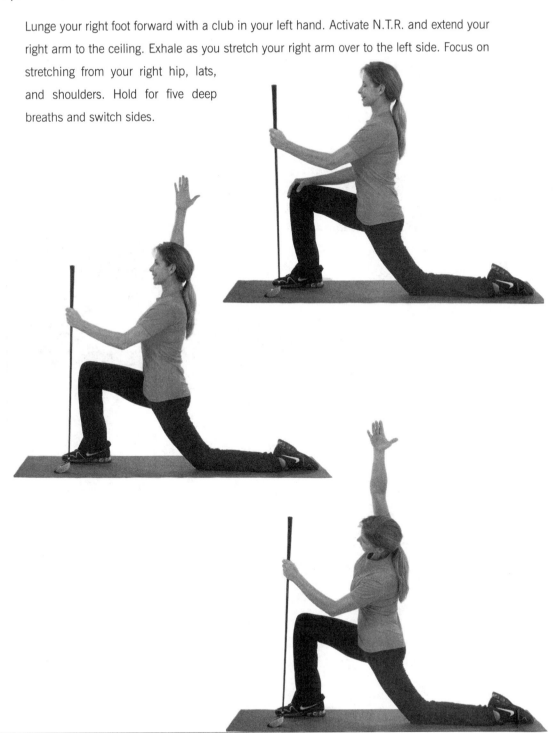

Dynamic Supine External Hip Stretch with Ball

Place your right foot on a stability ball and your left ankle outside your right knee. On your exhalation roll the ball toward you, focusing on the stretch in the left hip. Repeat five to ten times and switch sides.

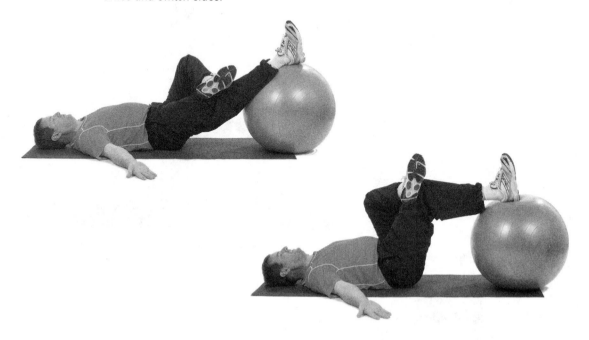

Glute Strengthener: Bridge Exercise with Leg Lifts

Lie on the ground and place your feet hip-width apart. Lift your hips off the floor. Keep the hips tucked without an excessive arch in your back. Hold for five breaths.

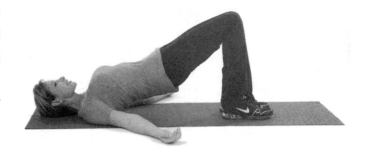

To make this more challenging, extend one leg at the same level as your opposite knee and hold for a count of ten. To increase the intensity, lift the extended leg up and down. Just remember to switch sides so both legs are worked equally.

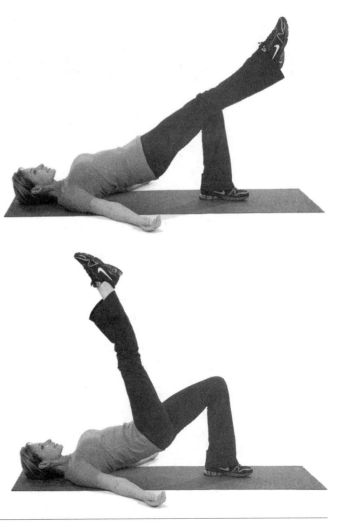

Groin Stretch

Sit with your back against a wall and the soles of your feet together. Bring your feet as close as possible to your groin and hold for three minutes.

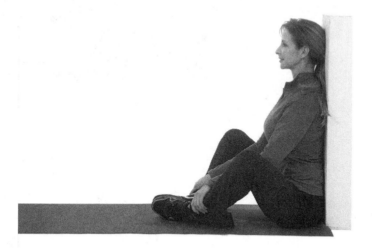

CHAPTER ELEVEN
COMING OVER THE TOP—SWING FLAW

In golf it's not who you are, what you are, or what you have that counts.

It's "How badly do you want to win?"

—BYRON NELSON

A CONSISTENT, REPEATABLE SWING path is elusive for many golfers. One of the most common swing flaws, particularly in higher-handicap golfers, is "coming over the top." This occurs when the upper body initiates the downswing instead of the lower body. This action creates an inconsistent swing path because the club is "thrown" outside the swing plane.

The main result of this swing flaw is improper sequencing, and it is essential for you to understand the importance of a proper sequence in your swing. When you come over the top, the lower body does not initiate the downswing and the result is a lack of power, poor ballstriking, and inconsistency. The lower body needs to participate in the kinetic link of the golf swing, but if you don't get it involved, the upper body will take over. Additionally, good balance, a proper weight shift, or weight transfer, and core strength will keep you from coming over the top.

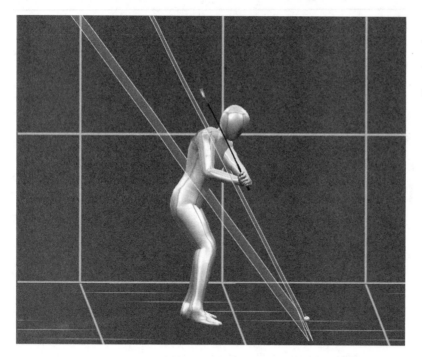

The golfer is coming over the top of the optimal swing path.

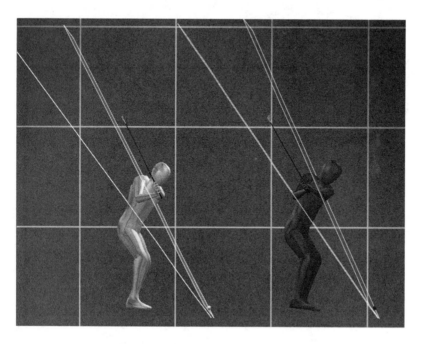

The golfer on the right brings the club within the proper swing plane.

PHYSICAL CAUSES OF COMING OVER THE TOP

Hip immobility

Lack of glute and lower-body strength

Trunk mobility

Shoulder mobility

Inefficient kinematic sequencing

HANK'S PERSPECTIVE

There are a few reasons why people come over the top. If a golfer takes the backswing too much to the inside in the takeaway they will almost surely swing the club over the top in the downswing. Another reason why golfers come over the top is that they don't have the movements of the golf swing in the proper sequence. If you fail to wind up or coil properly in the backswing, the downswing will almost surely start with the right shoulder leading the way, instead of the lower body. Ideally, the backswing builds a lot of coil so that the downswing starts down in a kind of automatic motion. The idea is for the lower body to resist turning as much as possible in the backswing and for the upper body to turn against the lower body's resistance. This creates coil, which is not unlike winding up a rubber band—the tighter the coil, the more automatic the unwinding, and this leads to power and proper timing through the downswing

FITNESS SOLUTIONS

Articulating Bridge Position

Bend your knees until your feet are approximately one foot from your glutes. Inhale as you press your lumbar spine toward the floor and engage the glutes. Exhale as you lift your hips off the floor, one vertebra at a time. Reverse the movement as you lower your glutes back to the floor. Repeat five to ten times.

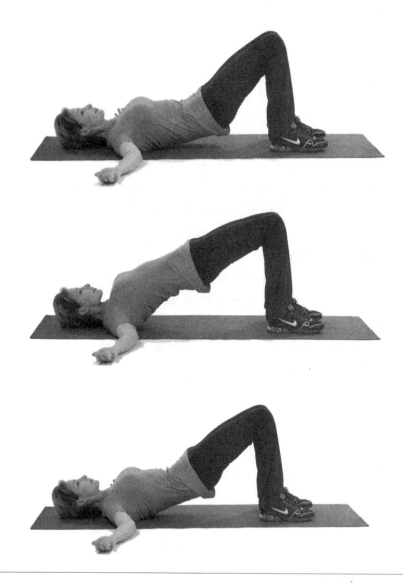

Standing Glute/Hip Stretch

Begin by placing your hands on a chair or a golf club to help you maintain your balance. Place your right ankle on the outside of your left knee. Inhale as you bend your left knee, sitting back as if you were sitting on a chair. Bring your chest toward your shin, rolling your shoulder blades together. Hold for three breaths and repeat five times. Switch sides.

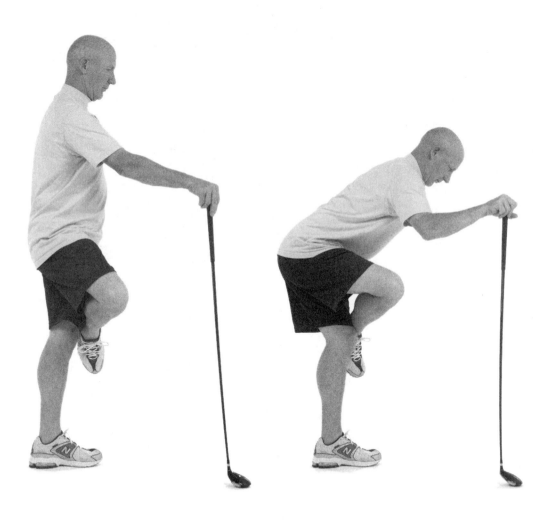

Dolphin Twist on Ball

Begin with your knees and triceps resting on a stability ball with your palms together. Stabilize your core by pulling your navel toward your spine. Bring your upper body parallel to the floor, focusing on the stretch in the lats and shoulders. Hold for three breaths. Stabilize your hips and rotate to the right, lifting your right arm off the ball. Switch sides and repeat five times in each direction.

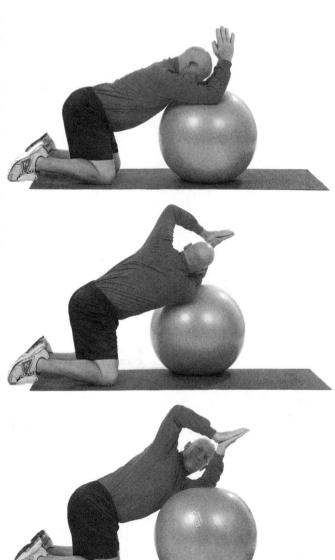

Spinal/Hip/Hamstring Series with Strap

Place a strap or belt around your right foot and extend your left leg. Flex both feet and activate both quads. Press your left hip toward the floor and extend your left arm perpendicular to your body. Hold for five breaths. Extend your right leg to the right, maintaining connection between your left glute and the floor. Hold for five breaths.

Place the strap in your left hand, extend your right arm perpendicular to your body, and bring your right leg and hip to the left. Hold for five breaths and switch sides.

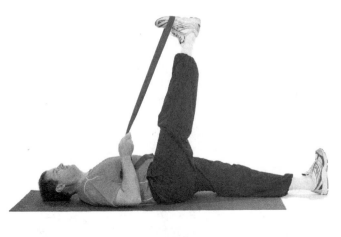

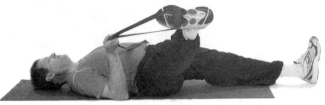

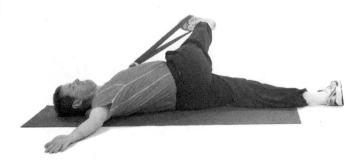

Alligator Twist with Shoulder Mobility

Place your right leg over your left knee. Rotate your spine and hips to the left, bringing the right arm perpendicular to your right shoulder.

Bring your right arm above your head. Hold for five breaths and switch sides.

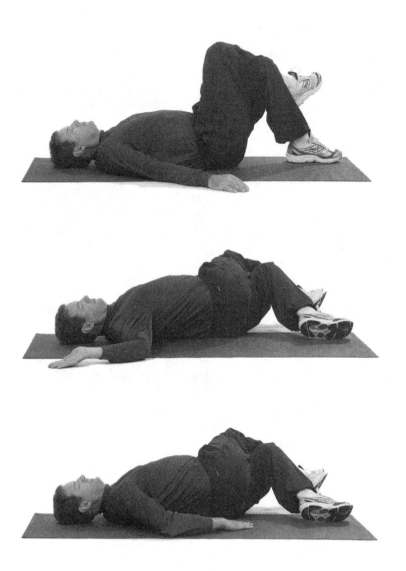

Trunk Stretch and Recoil Exercise

Place your left knee on the floor, with your right leg at a 90-degree angle. Place a club at chest height with your arms extended and stabilize your hips. Rotate your torso to the right and the left. Move with control, focusing on the range of motion in the trunk and stabilizing the hips. Repeat five times in each direction and switch sides.

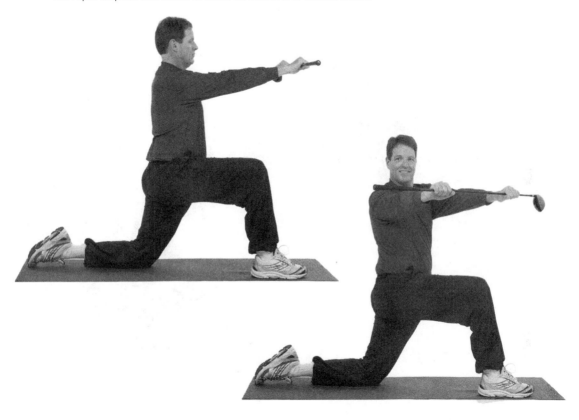

Glute Strengthener with Club and One Leg Extended

Lift your hips off the floor into a bridge position. Balance a club across your hips. Activate your left glute and extend your right leg at knee height. Hold for five to ten breaths while you keep your hips level. Switch sides.

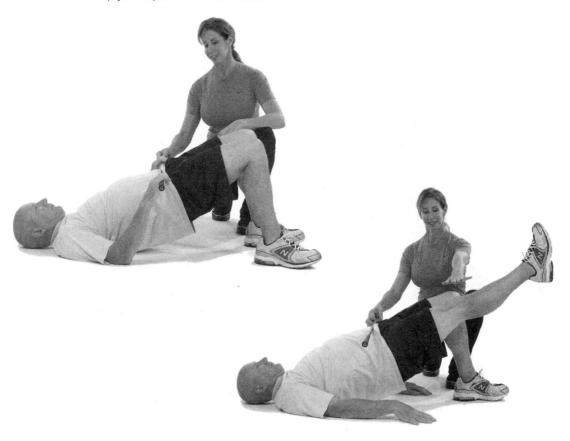

Full-Swing Drill

Rotate your hips, torso, and shoulders as if you were approaching the top of the backswing, initiating the downswing from your hips, and then bringing your torso and shoulders into a full finish position. Repeat five to ten times.

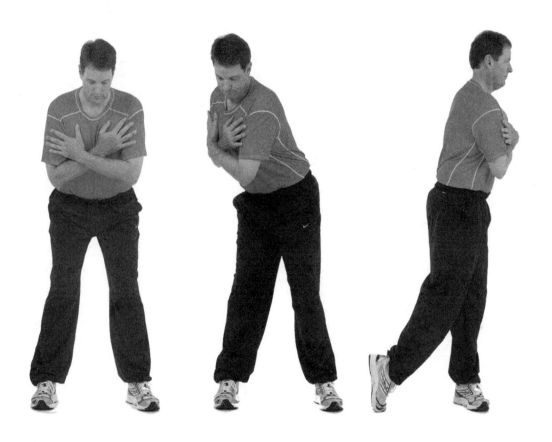

CHAPTER TWELVE
CASTING/SCOOPING THE BALL

Out here, it's just you and the ball.

—MIKE WEIR

CASTING, A COMMON swing flaw, is a breakdown in the swing during the downswing phase that occurs when the angle of the wrists is released too early. If the golfer is unable to maintain the proper wrist angle, the swing begins to resemble a fisherman casting his line. There is a related swing flaw called "scooping," which refers to a hand action in which the golfer attempts to scoop the ball off the ground. At the point of impact the clubhead reaches the ball before the proper angle of the hands and wrists. Note: Make sure to reread the information on wrist angles in Chapter Two.

It is obvious that strength in the hands, wrists, and forearms plays a role in casting, but the lower body is often to blame as well. Casting and scooping are by-products of the inefficient coiling of the spine in the backswing and lower-body action in the downswing. Improper balance and weight transfer can also lead to casting and scooping. As we have seen time and again, the lower body directly affects the upper-body function.

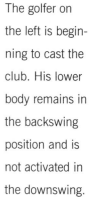

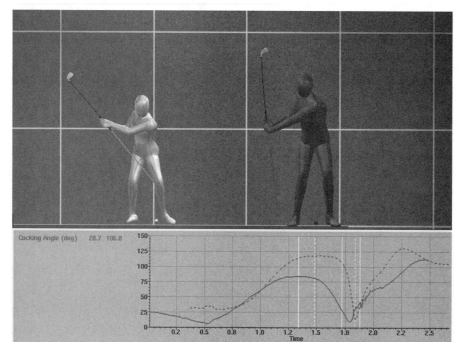

Cocking Angle (deg) 28.7 106.8

The golfer on the left is beginning to cast the club. His lower body remains in the backswing position and is not activated in the downswing.

The golfer on the right demonstrates proper wrist angle and position of the club shaft during the downswing. The golfer's lower body is active in the downswing.

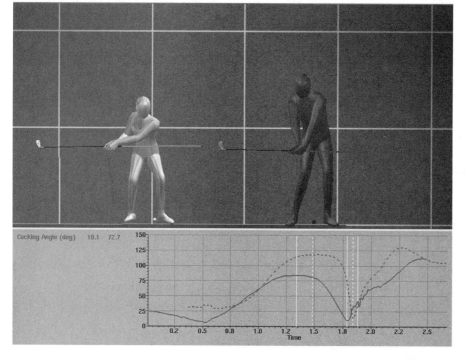

Cocking Angle (deg) 10.1 72.7

Note the incorrect position of the wrist on the golfer who exhibits casting. In addition, this golfer exhibits minimal lower-body activation.

PHYSICAL FIXES FOR CASTING

Create more mobility in the pelvis, specifically the ability to tilt the pelvis and initiate the lower body as the primary movement in the downswing

Generate more mobility in the internal rotators of the hips

Strengthen the glutes

Increase strength in the trunk

Develop more strength and flexibility in the hands and wrists

Develop proper balance and foot function

HANK'S PERSPECTIVE

There are a few reasons why golfers cast the club. The first is because they are trying to get the width necessary to get the club to come into the back of the ball properly. A golfer may also cast in order to shallow the club out if it is coming into the ball too steeply and headed into a collision with the ground. Finally, a casting motion is sometimes an attempt to get the golf club to square up faster. Ideally, a golfer should hold his release as long as he can so that the fastest point of the golf swing is right at the ball, but when you cast the club it reaches top speed before it gets to the ball. This holding of the release is often called delaying the hit. Again, a delayed hit is a more powerful and more repeatable way of releasing the golf club, as opposed to casting from the top of the swing. In order to delay the hit coming to the ball a player must start the downswing from the ground up; the first thing to move in the downswing are the feet. While the backswing starts from shoulders down, the downswing starts from the ground up, with the feet, the knees, and the hips. If the sequence is proper and well timed the result is a lagging of the golf club in the downswing, which results in a faster golf swing because the club whips into the ball. In order for all this to happen the proper coil must be built into the backswing and the lower body must initiate the downswing before the backswing is fully completed. This means that the golfer is momentarily going in two directions at once: backward with his shoulders while his feet, knees, and hips are moving forward.

FITNESS SOLUTIONS

Cat/Cow

Place your hands directly under your shoulders and your knees directly under your hips. Spread your fingers as wide as possible and press your entire hand into the floor. Inhale as you press your spine toward the floor and slightly lift your head, then exhale as you pull your navel toward your spine, engage your glutes, press your spine toward the ceiling, and tuck your chin into your chest. Now put the back of your hands on the floor and repeat ten times.

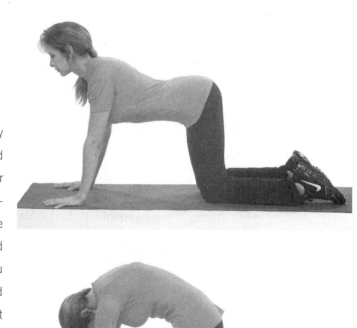

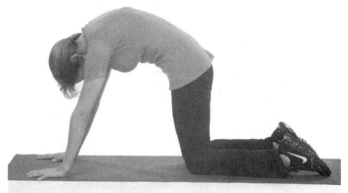

Seated Spinal Twist

Sit on the edge of a chair and elongate your spine by lifting your rib cage off your waist. Twist from your core, placing your right hand on your left knee and bringing your left arm to the back of the chair. Hold for five breaths and switch sides.

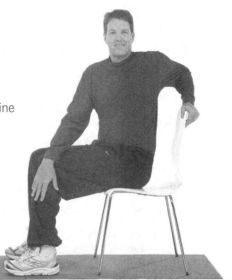

Spread-out Hand-to-Floor/Lat Stretch

Stand with your legs approximately four feet apart and rotate your legs and feet slightly inward. Reach your hands down to the seat of a chair. To make it more challenging, reach your hands all the way down to the ground, then reach them out to the right and left. Stretch your upper body to the right, focusing on the lat stretch. Hold for five breaths and switch sides.

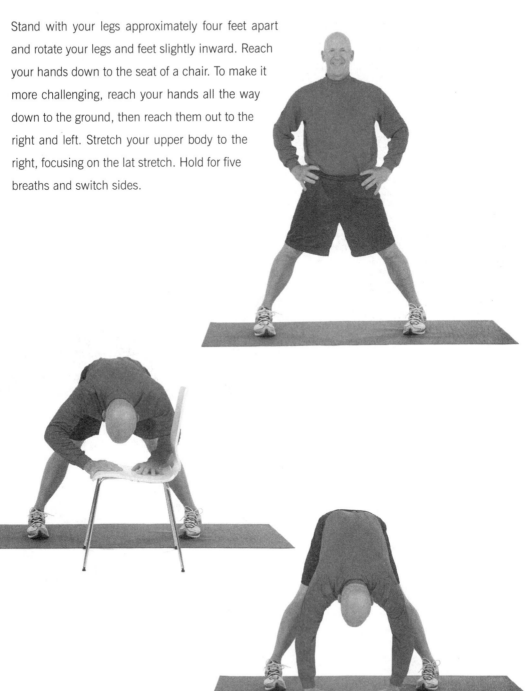

Supine Spinal/Hip Disassociation Stretch

Lie on your side and rest on your right shoulder, then bring your knees to a 90-degree angle. Note: Support your head and neck with a towel. Bring your arms to shoulder height, palms together. Maintain a connection between the knees. Inhale deeply, and on your exhale roll the upper body open, bringing the left arm as close to the floor as possible. Measure the distance from your left shoulder to the floor and measure the point at which your back immobility causes your knees to separate. Switch sides and repeat.

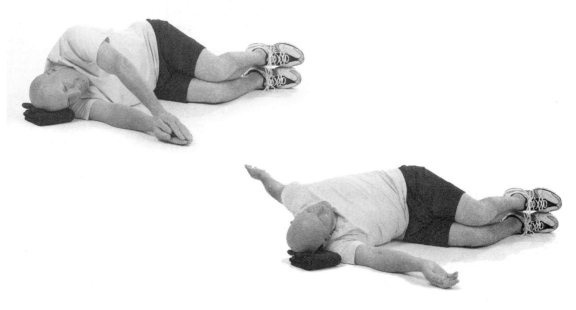

Core Crunch with Ball

Begin by lying on your back with your knees bent and your hands clasped behind your head to support your neck. Place a ball or towel between your knees. On your exhale, lift your chest off the floor. Repeat until you feel muscle fatigue. To make it more challenging, you can squeeze the upper and lower body together.

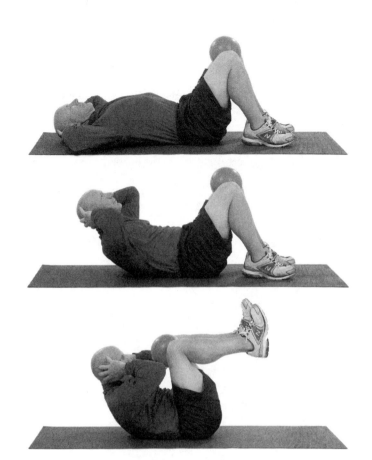

Extended Table

Begin on your hands and knees, activate your core, and then extend your right leg and left arm. Hold for five breaths and switch sides.

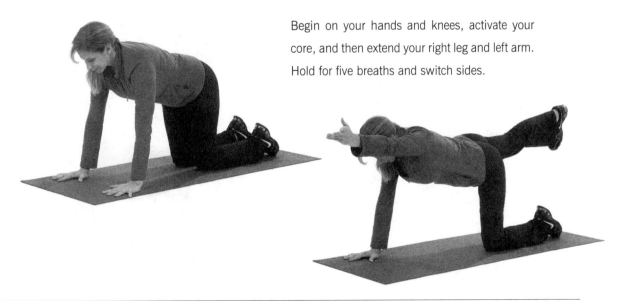

Superman

Lying facedown, extend your arms slightly wider than shoulder-width apart and your feet wider than hip-width apart. Exhale as you lift the opposite arm and leg. Hold for three breaths and switch sides. Repeat five times.

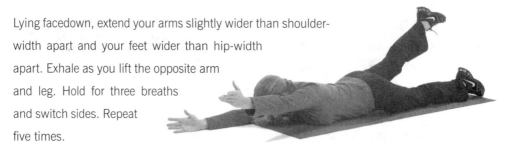

Power Turn Rotation with Club

Place the club at shoulder height. Lunge your left leg until your knee is at a 90-degree angle as you rotate your upper body to the left. Return to the starting position and switch sides. Repeat five times in each direction.

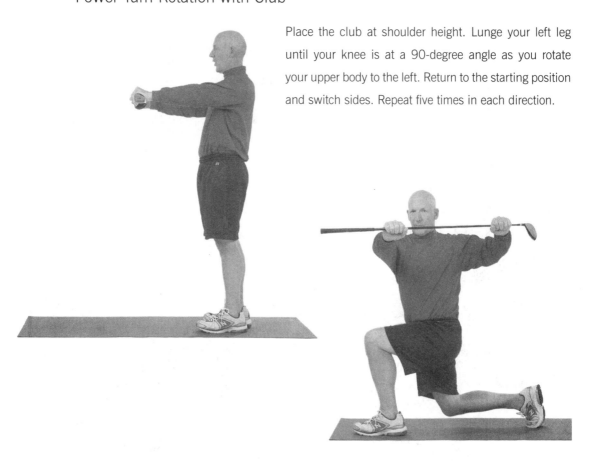

30-Second Speed Drill

Extend your left arm, support it with your right arm, and spread your fingers as wide as possible. Make a tight fist. Repeat as fast as possible for thirty seconds. Rest for one minute and repeat. Switch sides.

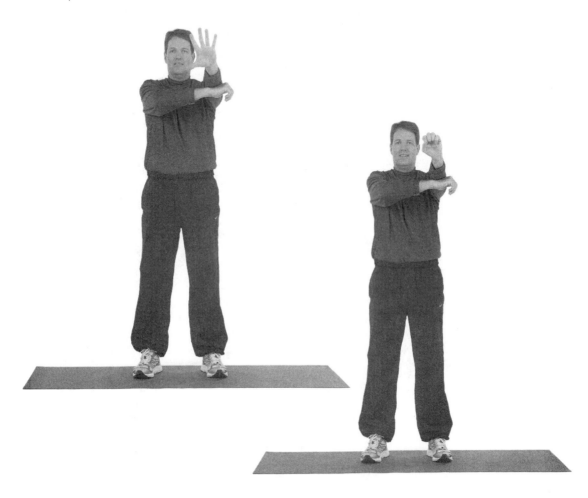

CHAPTER THIRTEEN
CHICKEN WING

Every golfer scores better when he learns his capabilities.

—TOMMY ARMOUR

I
N A SOLID golf shot the left arm remains extended past the point of impact. A breakdown in the left arm just past the point of impact is called a "chicken wing." You should see a golfer's clubhead before you see their elbow. If the golfer is chicken-winging, their left elbow will be visible at or just after the point of impact.

When the body is restricted in movement, either by a lack of flexibility (which is usually the case) or a lack of strength, extraneous or unnecessary movements occur in the golf swing. In the case of the chicken wing, a restriction in your shoulder turn causes an unnecessary and inefficient movement. With a chicken wing you'll experience a lack of power because the speed of the swing is compromised by the poor position of the left arm. The chicken wing can also cause "golfer's elbow."

Physically, a lack of lat, shoulder, and torso mobility contributes to this flaw. As far as strength is concerned, the musculature of the shoulders, specifically the rotators, will help you generate power. Strength in the hands, wrists, and forearms supports proper release and action in the hands. As with many of the upper-body swing flaws, developing an efficient lower-body swing sequence can help alleviate this flaw.

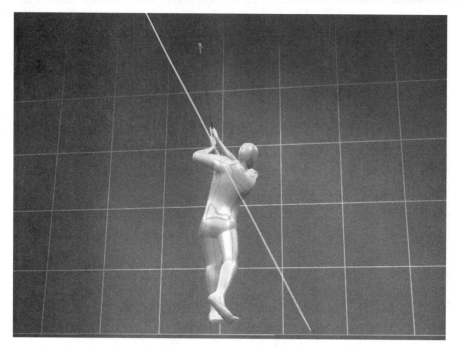

The golfer's chicken wing at the finish position is clearly evident in this image.

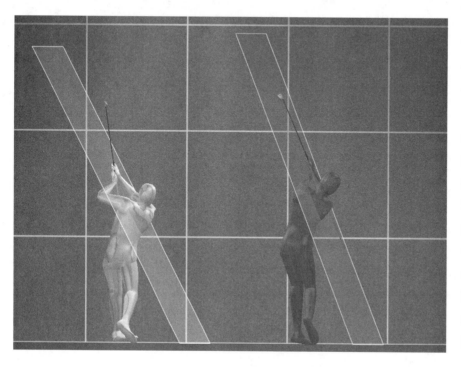

The golfer on the right exhibits the correct finish position with the arms extending toward the target and his hip rotation is in a more powerful position, while the golfer on the left exhibits chicken wing and less lower-body activation.

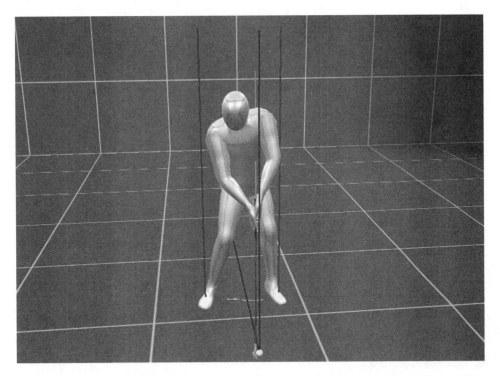

This golfer exhibits chicken wing at impact as well as at the finish position. His lower body exhibits little activation resulting in loss of power.

HANK'S PERSPECTIVE

With a chicken wing, the left arm bends instead of extending as the club is coming into impact. The results are a lack of power and often a lack of accuracy. The reason the accuracy is affected is because when the lead arm bends, it also stops rotating through the ball. The lack of continual rotation is a fundamental reason why more than 90 percent of all golfers slice the ball. One of the first things to check when a golfer slices his or her shots is the rotation of the clubface coming into impact. Instead of rotating the lead arm, which in turn squares the clubface, slicers reverse-rotate the clubface coming into the ball. Your arms need to rotate in the backswing to open the clubface, and they need to rotate in the downswing to bring the club onto the proper swing plane. This is called pronation in the backswing and supination in the downswing, and it's essential to squaring the clubface at impact.

FITNESS SOLUTIONS

Dynamic Internal/External Mobility from Twist

Cross your right leg over your left and place your left hand on your right knee. Rotate your body to the left, bringing your right arm to shoulder height. Inhale as you externally rotate your right shoulder, exhale as you internally rotate your right shoulder, bringing your right hand toward your waist. Repeat five to ten times and switch sides.

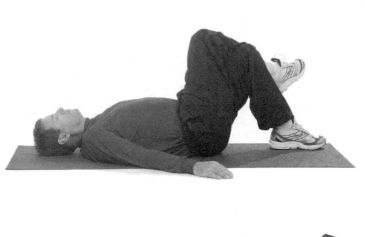

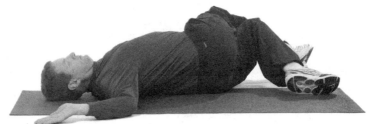

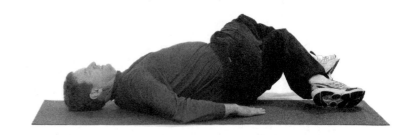

Twisting Table

Get down on all fours and place your right elbow behind your head. Inhale and twist from the thoracic spine toward the ceiling. Exhale and tuck your right shoulder under your left shoulder. Repeat five times and hold for five more breaths.

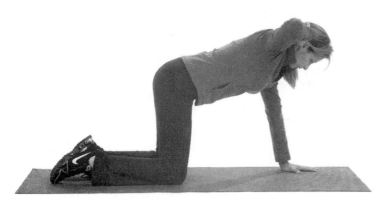

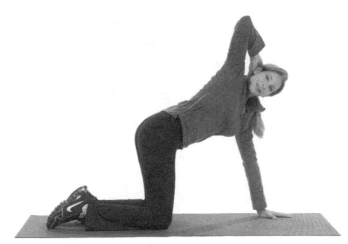

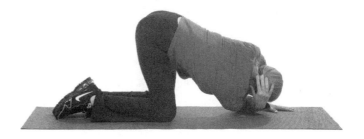

Shoulder Stretch with Club Behind Back

Place a club or towel in your right hand and bring the arm over your head and behind your back. Bring your left arm behind your back and clasp the club or towel. Inhale as you gently pull, then exhale and release. Repeat five times and switch arms.

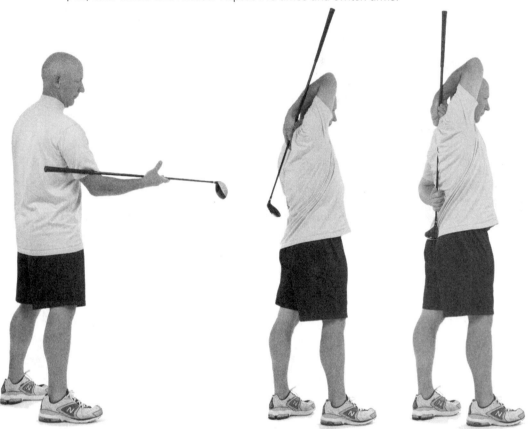

Clockwork/Shoulder Mobility Exercises

Stand with your body touching a wall, then slightly bend the knees and internally rotate your legs and feet. Point your thumbs toward the ceiling, reaching your arms above your head. Lower your shoulders away from your ears and press your arms back, focusing on muscle activation in the mid-back. Hold for five breaths. Bring your arms to a 45-degree angle. Hold for five breaths. Bring your arms to shoulder height. Hold for five breaths.

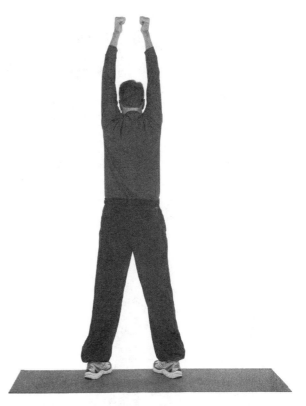

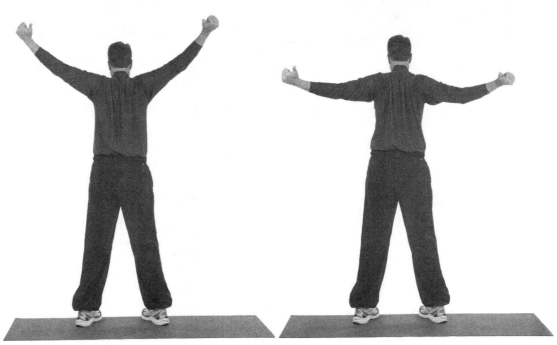

Hand, Wrist, and Forearm Series with Club

Place a club in your palm. Roll your wrist and forearm open, then roll your wrist closed, toward the floor. Extend your hand toward the floor, and then cock the wrist back toward you. Repeat five times and switch sides.

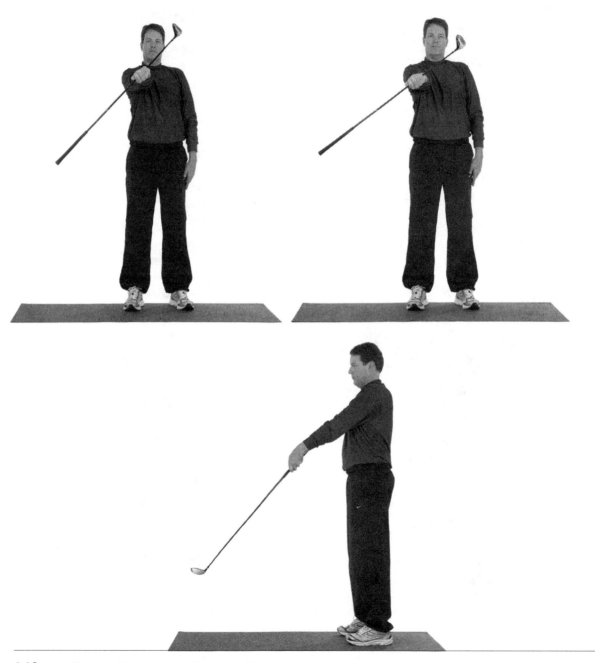

Rear Delt Exercises on the Ball

Place a stability ball under your hips. Squeeze your legs together to stabilize the lower body. Lift your chest off the ball, with your thumbs facing the ceiling and your arms extended slightly wider than shoulder-width apart. Lift the arms five to ten times. Rest for one minute. Next bring your arms perpendicular to your shoulders. Lift the arms five to ten times. Rest for one minute. Lastly, bring your arms to a 45-degree angle, thumbs facing the ceiling. Lift the arms five to ten times. Rest for one minute.

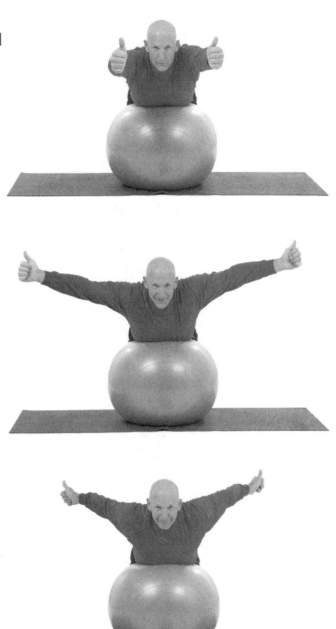

XYZ Balance Rotation Drill with Club

Extend your left leg onto a stability ball and extend your arms and club to shoulder height. Inhale, activating N.T.R., and rotate your torso over your left leg. Repeat three times and switch sides.

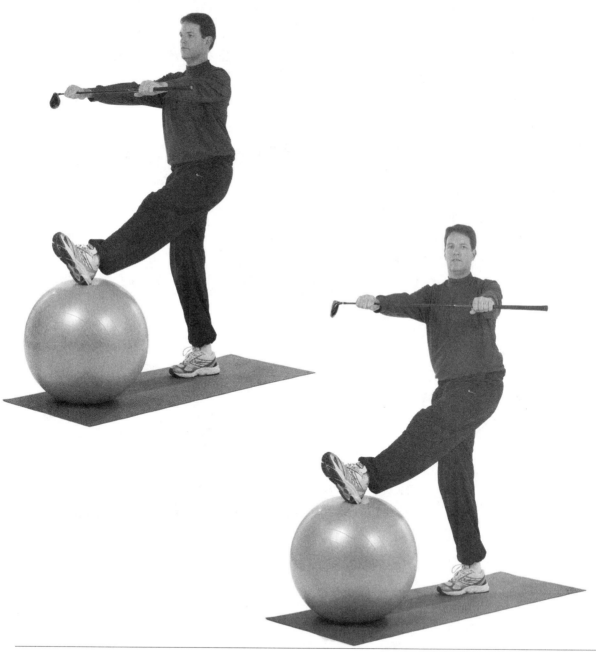

CHAPTER FOURTEEN
REVERSE "C" SPINE ANGLE

Why is it twice as difficult to hit a ball over water than over sand?

—AUTHOR UNKNOWN

A T ONE OF my golf performance centers I noticed a gentleman warming up, hitting off the launch monitor. He was in his early fifties, very tall with a powerful upper body. His clubhead speed was above normal but his distance off the tee was not consistent with his power. His finish position was less than optimal, with a minimal hip extension that left him significantly off-balance. I approached and told him that I could help him gain fifteen yards off the tee. Although initially skeptical, he agreed to a quick physical assessment. I uncovered significant hip-mobility and core-stability problems. I prescribed seven exercises targeting the core, lower-body flexibility, and strength exercises. In addition, he committed to six weekly lessons to work on his mechanics. To date, he is regularly driving the ball farther, getting the distance I promised, and hitting more consistent golf shots.

Immediately following impact, the follow-through phase of the swing begins.

In basic terms, the follow-through may be thought of as a mirror image of the backswing, although each player has his or her unique follow-through. Ideally, the follow-through should be a well-balanced, upright posture. When your upper body bends backward and/or bends laterally during the follow-through, you have what's called a "reverse C" swing fault. We should note that a small reverse "C" is acceptable, but an excessive amount places disproportionate force on the lumbar spine, causing strain and injury. Additionally, the reverse "C" creates a finish position that is out of balance and not fully extended toward the target. Primarily a result of poor core strength and hip mobility, the reverse "C" is perhaps one of the easiest swing flaws to alleviate.

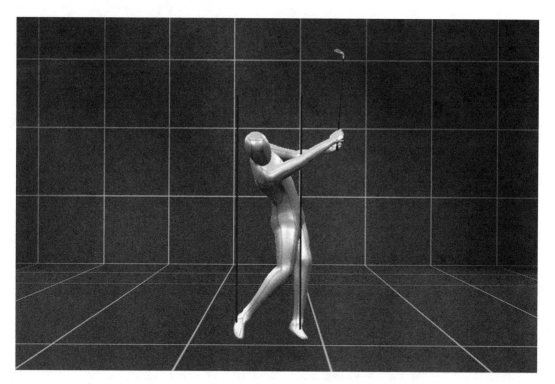

The golfer is beginning to exhibit the reverse "C" position through impact. Note the excessive bend in his torso.

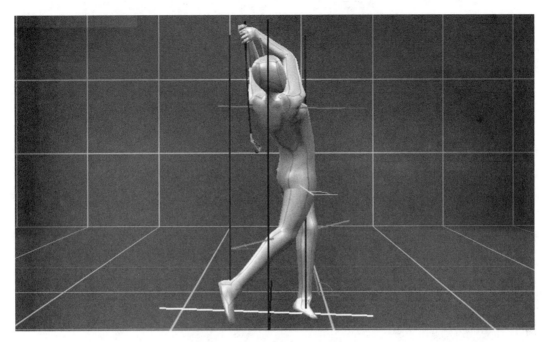

The classic reverse "C" position in the finish position. Note the compression in his lumber spine and back-bending motion of his upper back and head.

HANK'S PERSPECTIVE

The more a player finishes with a reverse "C" the more a player will hook the ball and at the same time put stress on the lower back. It is interesting to note that younger, more flexible golfers tend to finish with more of a reverse "C" coming into and through the ball. As we get older and lose flexibility it becomes harder to finish with any reverse "C" to speak of. Your back should be arched at least a little bit as you come through the ball—this helps to ensure that you are hitting from the inside and that you finish on balance—so it is essential that as a golfer you at least have enough flexibility to have a little reverse "C" coming into the ball. This is probably the biggest change in the so-called modern swing of today—in years past players would swing and finish with a bigger reverse "C" than they do today. Too much of reverse "C" is caused by the head and upper body dropping back as the club approaches impact. This mistake causes the body to slow down relative to the club and makes the clubface close too rapidly, invariably resulting in a hook.

FITNESS SOLUTIONS

Spinal Rotation with Arms Perpendicular to the Body

Inhale as you bring your legs to the right, keeping your shoulders in contact with the floor. Then exhale, initiating the movement from your oblique abdominal muscles, and bring the legs back to the starting position. Switch sides and repeat ten times in each direction. To make this more challenging, lift your legs off the floor, with your knees at a 90-degree angle.

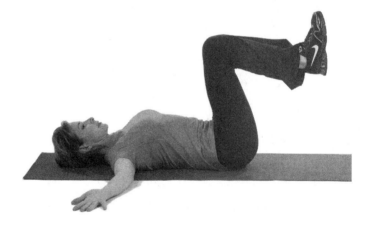

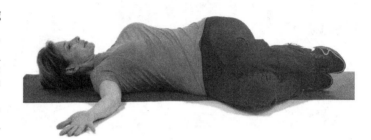

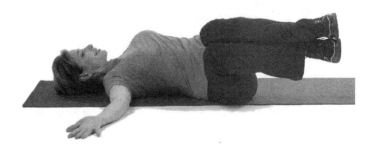

Pilates Roll-downs

Squeeze a stability ball between your hands. Inhale as you articulate your spine down to the floor. When your bottom rib touches the floor, exhale and roll back to the starting position. Repeat ten to twenty times.

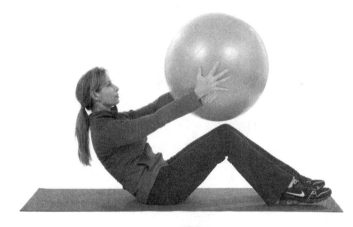

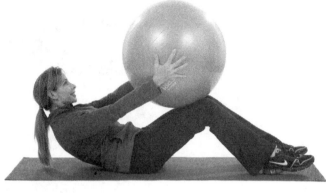

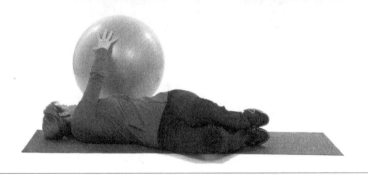

The Turn

Begin on your back with your knees bent, feet on the floor, and a stability ball in your hands. Inhale as you roll your arms to the left and your legs to the right. Exhale as you return to the starting position. Make sure you initiate the movement from your oblique abdominals. Switch sides and repeat five times.

Core Crunch with Ball

Begin by lying on your back with your knees bent and your hands clasped behind your head to support your neck. Place a ball or towel between your knees. On your exhale, lift your chest off the floor. Repeat until you feel muscle fatigue. To make it more challenging, you can squeeze the upper and lower body together.

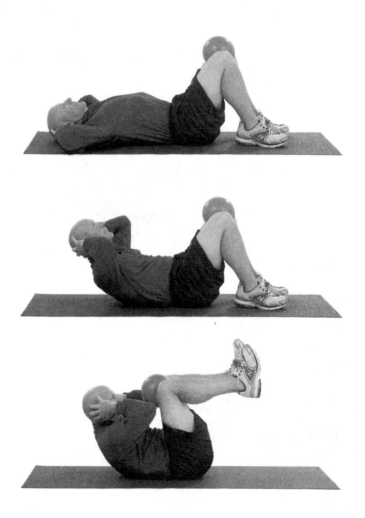

Modified Cobra

Begin with your hands placed next to your chest, your legs together, and the tops of your feet on the floor. Inhale as you squeeze your legs together, activating the glutes. Exhale as you lift your chest off the floor. Repeat dynamically five times. Hold for five more breaths, and focus on activating the rhomboid muscles. Keep your shoulders moving down, away from your ears.

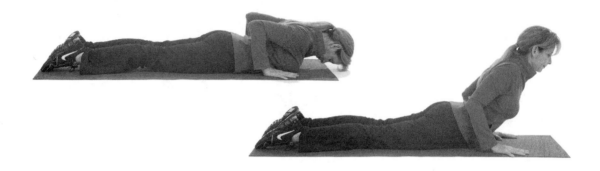

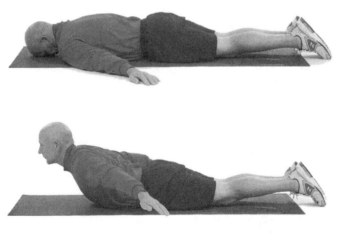

Locust

Place your hands next to your body with your legs together. Lift your legs and upper body off the floor. Hold for three deep breaths, then relax. Repeat three times.

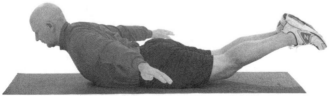

SECTION THREE

THE ROBERTS FLEX-FIT METHOD FOR A STRONGER BODY AND LOWER SCORES

CHAPTER FIFTEEN
BUILD YOUR BACK STRENGTH

You swing your best when you have the fewest things to think about.

—BOBBY JONES

I RECEIVE THOUSANDS OF e-mails from golfers regarding golf performance, injury prevention, and mental conditioning. Overwhelmingly, most of the questions I receive are about back pain.

The golf swing places a repetitive strain on the body and tremendous pressure on the lumbar spine, often causing back pain. Off the course, back pain contributes to more lost work days and painkiller consumption than any other physical complaint. During the swing your spine will experience shear, compression, and rotational forces—roughly a hundred times per round! Concentrating your golf fitness program on the health of your spine is critical for power, distance, and consistency, as well as longevity in the game.

It is important to understand that many factors affect your back. Hip function is one of the most critical components of efficient movement. Healthy hips affect the lower back and your shoulder mobility, and they give you the best opportunity for an efficient kinematic sequence. A complete back program includes the following components:

- Core strength
- Hip function
- Hamstring flexibility
- Lumbar-spine flexibility and strength
- Proper posture

FITNESS SOLUTIONS

Pelvic Tilts

Begin on your back with your knees bent and your feet flat on the floor. Inhale, bringing the lumbar spine into a neutral position. Exhale as you press your lower back toward the floor and tilt your pelvis toward the ceiling. Repeat ten times.

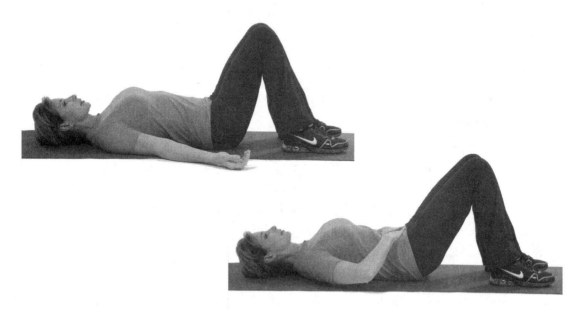

Knees to Chest

Inhale as you bring your arms above your head. Exhale as you pull your left knee to your chest and your head to your knee. Switch sides and repeat ten times.

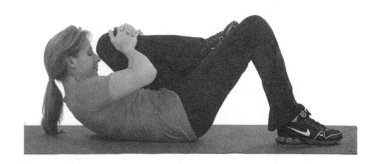

Dynamic Window Washers—Internal/External Hip Stretch

Begin with your feet wider than hip-width apart. Inhale as you bring both knees to the right, then exhale as you return to the starting position. Switch sides and repeat five times in each direction.

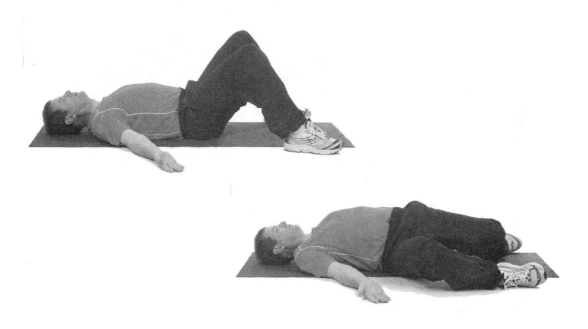

Cat/Cow Spinal Warm-up

Place your hands directly under your shoulders and your knees directly under your hips. Spread your fingers as wide as possible and press your entire hand into the floor. Inhale as you press your spine toward the floor and slightly lift your head, then exhale as you pull your navel toward your spine, engage your glutes, press your spine toward the ceiling, and tuck your chin into your chest. Repeat ten times.

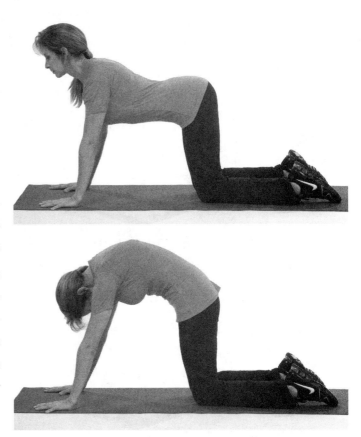

Articulating Bridge Position

Bend your knees until your feet are approximately one foot from your glutes. Inhale as you press your lumbar spine toward the floor and engage the glutes. Exhale as you lift your hips off the floor, one vertebra at a time. Reverse the movement as you lower your glutes back to the floor. Repeat five to ten times.

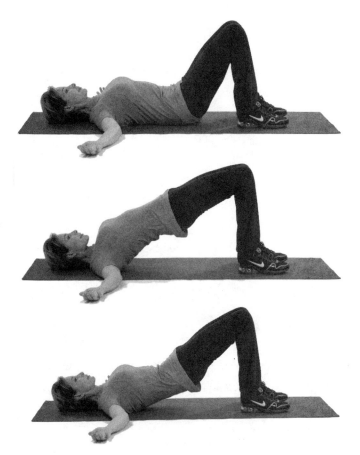

Modified Cobra

Begin with your hands placed next to your chest, with your legs together and the tops of your feet on the floor. Inhale as you squeeze your legs together, activating the glutes. Exhale as you lift your chest off the floor. Repeat dynamically five times. Hold for five more breaths, and focus on activating the rhomboid muscles. Keep your shoulders moving down, away from your ears.

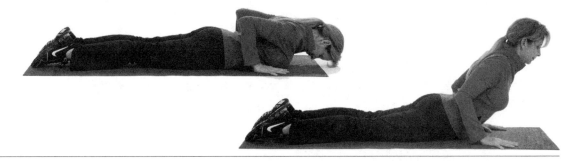

Extended Table

Begin on your hands and knees, activate your core, and extend your right leg and left arm. Hold for five breaths and switch sides.

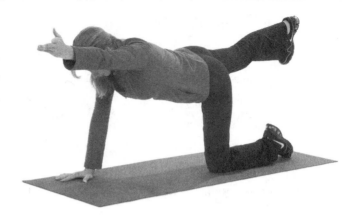

Superman

Lying facedown, extend your arms slightly wider than shoulder-width apart and your feet wider than hip-width apart. Exhale as you lift the opposite arm and leg. Hold for three breaths and switch sides. Repeat five times.

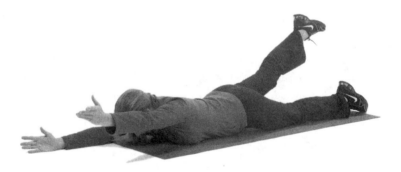

Spinal/Hip/Hamstring Series with Strap

Place a strap or belt around your right foot and extend your left leg. Flex both feet and activate both quads. Press your left hip toward the floor and extend your left arm perpendicular to your body. Hold for five breaths. Extend your right leg to the right, maintaining connection between your left glute and the floor. Hold for five breaths.

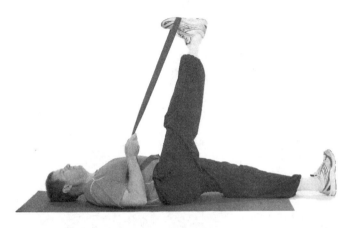

Place the strap in your left hand, extend your right arm perpendicular to your body, and bring your right leg and hip to the left. Hold for five breaths and switch sides.

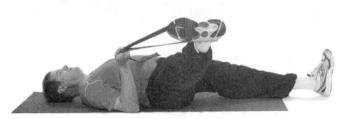

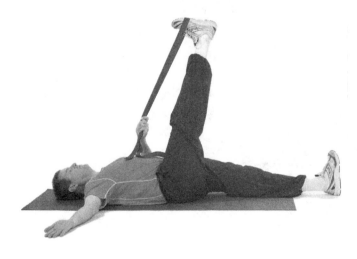

Legs up the Wall Groin Stretch

Bring your glutes up against a wall, placing your legs up the wall and your body on the floor. Place a towel under your head if your neck is hyperextended. Rest in this position for three to five minutes. Bring the soles of your feet together and bring your feet toward your groin. Rest in this position for an additional three to five minutes.

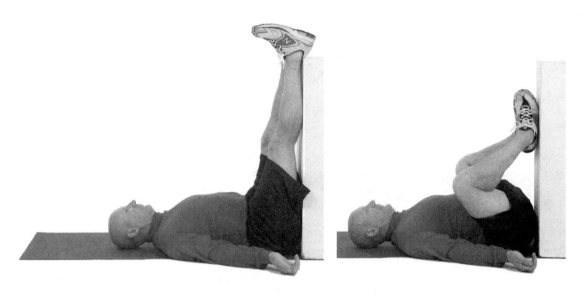

Passive Supine Spinal Rotation with Support

Cross your left leg over your right leg, place your arms perpendicular to your body, and rotate your lower body to the right. Place a towel under your knees and rest in this position for three to five minutes. Breathe deeply and allow your body to move deeper. Switch sides.

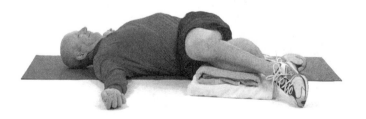

CHAPTER SIXTEEN
CORE STABILITY AND STRENGTH—
THE FUNDAMENTAL
OF GOLF FITNESS

Golf is deceptively simple and endlessly complicated; it satisfies the
soul and frustrates the intellect. It is at the same time rewarding and
maddening—and it is without a doubt the greatest game mankind has
ever invented.

—ARNOLD PALMER

CORE CONDITIONING HAS become a buzzword in fitness, but what exactly is it
and how will developing a strong, stable core benefit your game? The core
refers to all the anterior and posterior muscles of the torso: rectus abdominis, internal and external obliques, transverse abdominis, erector spinae, and glutes.

In the golf swing the core stabilizing muscles are active in the address position and increase activation during the takeaway phase of the swing. Core stability

helps you maintain balance, strike the ball consistently, and increase your rotational speed, thus maximizing your clubhead speed and leaving you in a balanced finish position. The repetitive movement of the golf swing requires core strength, and the ability to stabilize the core during the swing helps you maintain a consistent spine angle and reduce many swing flaws. If you are looking for more power and a more consistent swing plane you must work the core. Harnessing your power requires a coiling and uncoiling of the spine, and this action is more easily accomplished with a flexible, stable, and strong core.

FITNESS SOLUTIONS: CORE FLEXIBILITY SERIES

Pelvic Tilts

With your knees bent and your feet flat on the floor, inhale and bring your lower back into a neutral position. Exhale as you press your lower back toward the floor and tilt your pelvis toward the ceiling. Repeat ten times.

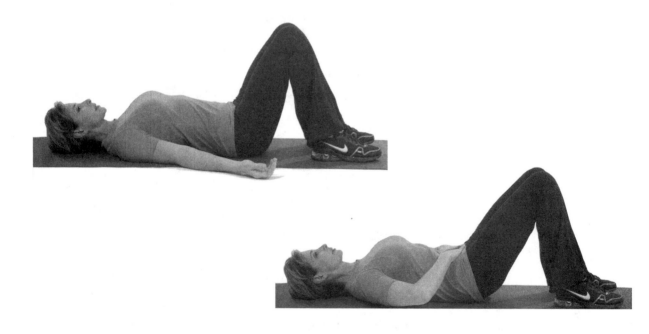

Articulating Bridge Position

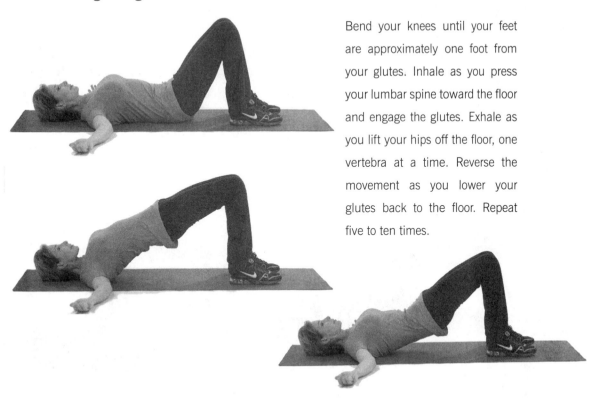

Bend your knees until your feet are approximately one foot from your glutes. Inhale as you press your lumbar spine toward the floor and engage the glutes. Exhale as you lift your hips off the floor, one vertebra at a time. Reverse the movement as you lower your glutes back to the floor. Repeat five to ten times.

TVA Abdominal Lift Exercise

Place your hands on your knees and create a posterior tilt in the pelvis. Inhale deeply and exhale all the air out of the lungs. Hold the air out and "snap" or pull your navel into your spine. Hold for three seconds, release the TVAs (the lower abdominals), and inhale deeply again. Take five normal breaths and repeat three times.

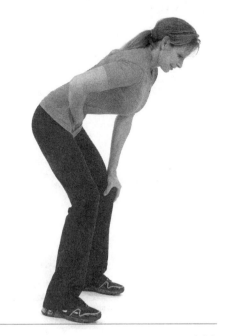

Cat/Cow Spinal Warm-up

Place your hands directly under your shoulders and your knees directly under your hips. Spread your fingers as wide as possible and press your entire hand into the floor. Inhale as you press your spine toward the floor and slightly lift your head, then exhale as you pull your navel toward your spine, engage your glutes, press your spine toward the ceiling, and tuck your chin into your chest. Repeat ten times.

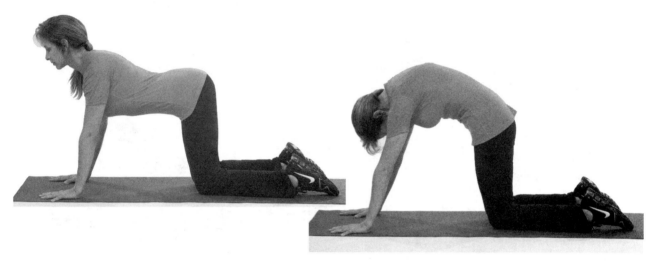

Extended Side Stretch

Place your left hand, knee, and right foot in a straight line. Press your foot into the floor and pull your navel toward your spine. Inhale deeply and stretch your right arm over your head. Hold for five to seven deep breaths and switch sides. The more you tuck your pelvis under, the more you will feel the stretch.

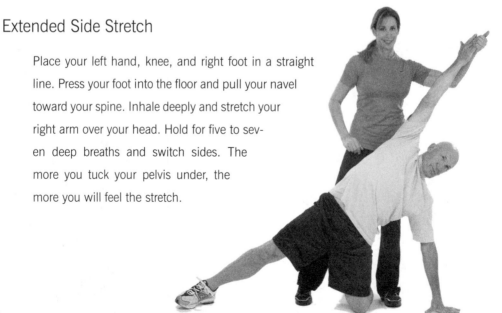

Core-Strengthening Series

Begin on your back, with your knees bent and a towel between your hands. Press your navel to your spine, while your lower back and rib cage remain connected to the floor. Lift your right foot one inch off the floor. Slowly switch sides. To make this more challenging, you can bring your left leg off the floor with your knee at a 90-degree angle while you extend your right leg off the floor. On your exhalation, switch sides. Repeat five times.

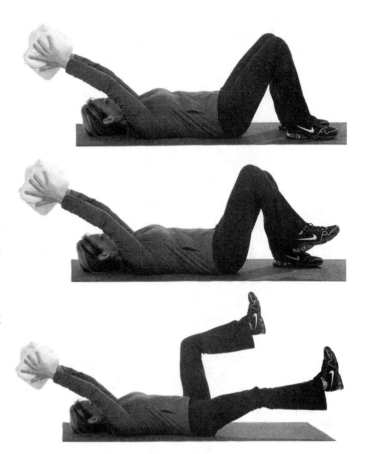

Pilates Roll Downs

Squeeze a stability ball between your hands. Inhale as you articulate your spine down to the floor. When your bottom rib touches the floor, exhale and roll back to the starting position. Repeat ten to twenty times.

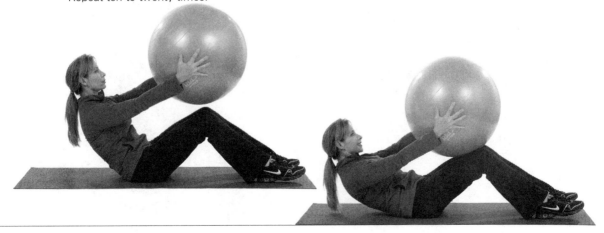

Core Crunch with Ball

Begin by lying on your back with your knees bent and your hands clasped behind your head to support your neck. Place a ball or towel between your knees. On your exhale, lift your chest off the floor. Repeat until you feel muscle fatigue. To make it more challenging, you can squeeze the upper and lower body together.

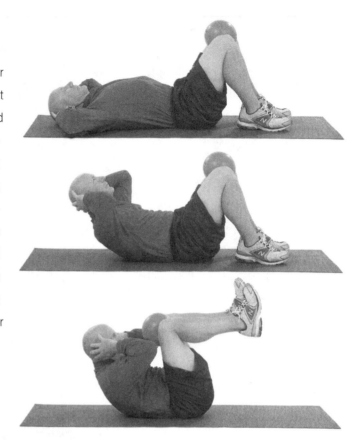

Extended Table with Abdominal Crunch

Begin on all fours and stabilize your core. Inhale as you extend your left arm and right leg. Lift the leg and arm as high as possible without arching your back. Exhale as you pull your left elbow to your right knee. Repeat five to ten times. Hold the left arm and right leg extended for thirty seconds and switch sides.

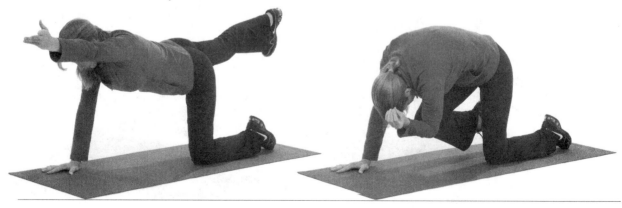

Modified Cobra

Begin with your hands placed next to your chest, with your legs together and the tops of your feet on the floor. Inhale as you squeeze your legs together, activating the glutes. Exhale as you lift your chest off the floor. Repeat dynamically five times. Hold for five more breaths and focus on activating the rhomboid muscles. Keep your shoulders moving down, away from your ears.

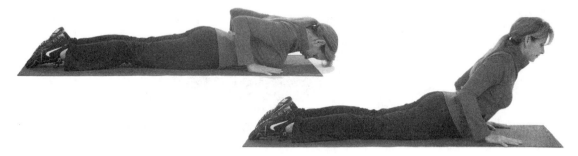

Plank

Place your hands directly under your shoulders, spread your fingers wide, and press your palms into the floor. Maintain a stable plank position without letting your back sag for thirty seconds to one minute. Repeat three times.

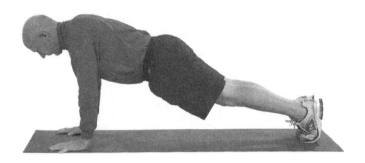

Side Plank

Place your forearm directly under your shoulder, with your feet stacked and your balance resting on the outside edge of your foot. Activate your oblique abdominals and lift your hips off the floor. Hold for thirty seconds. Repeat three times.

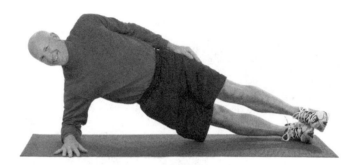

Power Oblique Crunch on Ball

Place the ball under your right hip, left leg placed over the right as you brace your lower body against the wall. Bring your hands behind your head and stretch the left side. Hold for five breaths. Inhale deeply and on your exhalation crunch your upper body, lifting your left elbow toward your left hip. Repeat ten to twenty times and switch sides.

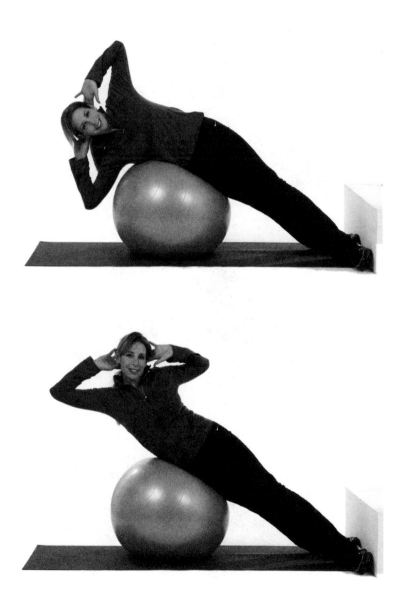

Power Hip Lift/Glute Strengthener on Ball

Place the ball under your heels and pull your navel toward your spine. Inhale as you activate your glutes, exhale as you lift your hips off the floor. Repeat ten times and rest for one minute.

Lift your hips off the floor and on your exhale roll the ball away from your body, focusing on keeping your hips lifted off the floor. Repeat five to ten times.

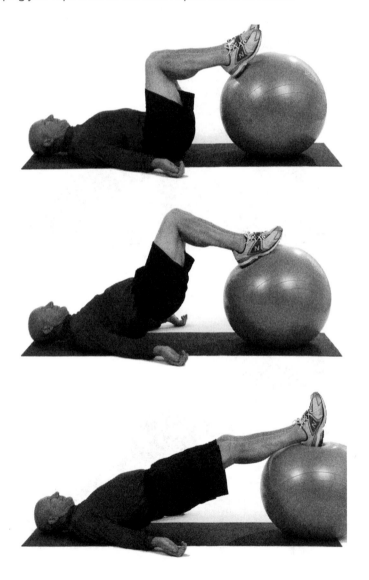

CHAPTER SEVENTEEN
BALANCE, PROPRIOCEPTION, VISION, AND FOOT FUNCTION

I like my ankles to be free, which is why I play in shoes and not boots.

—HARRY VARDON

GOOD BALANCE IS the ability to maintain our center of gravity and the ability to control the position of our body, whether we're standing still or moving. What is a balanced swing? We should be balanced at address, with proper weight distribution, good knee flexion, and an athletic stance. From this balanced static position we can then transfer to the dynamic phase of the swing, from the takeaway to the finish position.

There are three components that effect balance: the eyes, the inner ear, and something called proprioception. Proprioception is the coordination of the limbs and body position via the reception of stimuli by the nervous system. Without the proper function of these three components, along with healthy foot function, the golfer's swing mechanics will be poor.

Dr. Debbie Crews, author of *Golf: Energy in Motion*, describes the complexity of golf and the mind/body connection:

"The more complex the task, the longer the programming time. Longer programming time takes place behind the ball. Movement is coordinated relative to the whole swing, not to the thousands of individual movements that make up that swing. The mind, brain, and body plan the motion; joint angles and muscle torques follow. Focusing on moving the handle of the club through space in the desired path, rather than focusing on the actual movement of the body itself, can be very effective. If the swing is finished in balance facing the target, many components of the swing had to fall into place without the golfer having to focus on each one separately."

Practicing balance-conditioning exercises and executing complex movements on an uneven surface or on one leg facilitates proprioception. Additionally, moving in and out of a specific exercise with purposeful awareness of the placement of the feet facilitates proprioception. For example, lifting one leg off the floor and placing the foot back in exact position develops an awareness of where your body is in space.

VISION

The following information is provided by Dr. Alan Reichow, Nike's global research director for vision science, and director of research and development for Nike SST™. Dr. Reichow has researched the role of vision in sport, and provided comprehensive diagnostic, remedial, and enhancement vision care services to thousands of professional and amateur athletes, including elite golfers, for the past thirty-two years.

It was identified earlier in this chapter that "there are three components that affect balance—the eyes, the inner ear, and something called proprioception." You will note the order she listed these skills. "The eyes," or a broader and more encompassing term, "vision," is the dominant human sense.

The phrase "the eyes lead the body" was coined by the late American Football's Cleveland Browns Coach Blanton Collier in the 1950s. He observed that the best players in certain positions were the ones that popped their head and eyes toward their final goal. These five simple words have served as the basis for the vision performance research and clinical care of athletes I have been involved with over the past thirty-two years. For most, the "eyes" simply are related to how clearly one sees. Certainly, this is an important component, but the "eyes" are merely the gateway to a complex visual system we rely on for interpreting the world around us and making appropriate and timely responses. Balance is a common denominator across all of these visually driven responses.

In the world of sport we all have those moments of greatness. It just so happens that the best of the best display those moments of greatness routinely. They are consistently at a high level. Specific to golf, we all recall those occasions of reading a challenging thirty-foot breaking putt and dropping it. Or the approach shot with hazards seemingly everywhere, where we leave ourselves with a short birdie. What's the magic to putting these performances together more often? A critical, but often neglected aspect of elite human performance is vision.

Whether it's the baseball player who is in a hot batting streak or the golfer who is seemingly dropping every putt, most athletes experiencing such a consistent high level of performance make such reference as "I'm 'seeing' the ball or line well."

There are three basic questions that we look at relative to "seeing it well":

1. What does "seeing it well" mean?
2. How can we test for "seeing it well"?
3. How can we provide the tools or training so that an athlete can turn the "seeing it well" switch on whenever she or he wants?

This section of the chapter will take an introductory look at these questions and will provide some guidance to the golfer in how to begin influencing "seeing it well," with particular emphasis on balance.

Vision involves collection of the light information of the world around us through our eyes, the most sophisticated cameras ever created. That information is then transmitted primarily to the visual cortex, and to a lesser extent, other areas of our brain, where it is processed, resulting in a motor response. Humans possess two eyes for a purpose. These two eyes operate on a summation premise in that the power (or quality) of the visual signal we utilize is stronger and more accurate with the combination of the two eyes together. Relative to skills such as depth perception, spatial awareness, and balance, two-eye use is definitely more powerful than one-eyed use. Given normal two-eye use, it is critical to keep the two eyes on the object of regard as much as possible.

Vision/Balance Relationship Exercise #1

This drill will demonstrate the importance of two-eye use on depth perception and balance.

While standing on one foot with one eye closed, toss a coin high into the air, with your dominant hand out in front of your body. While it is in flight, pat your stomach with your dominant hand and then reach out for the catch. Next, repeat the process with both eyes open. Most individuals, unless you have a significant two-eye use limitation, will experience much greater accuracy of catching and stability with two-eye use.

Each of your eyes transmits approximately 1.1 million nerve fibers to the central nervous system, with nearly ten percent to balance control. How powerful is vision as compared to the inner year, you might ask? In most healthy individuals vision will override the vestibular and proprioceptive systems in balance and stability if there is disagreement. As an example, you may have been to an amusement park fun house with a room painted to simulate a dramatic tilt to the right or left. Virtually all who experience this will feel the strong pull toward the lower corner of the simulated room. In this case, the vestibular and proprioceptive syetems are saying that everything is "cool," but the visual system is screaming that all is not well and you'll feel the drift to the side. Similarly, you may have been sitting in an Omnitype theater watching simulated high-speed action as in a jet or high-performance car traveling through a maze of sharp turns. Once again, although the vestibular and proprioceptive information is stable, the visual system is communicating a wild ride, that is "felt" by most people. For some individuals, the power of the signal is so strong, that they may experience slight discomfort or even nausea. In most real world situations though, the visual, vestibular, and proprioceptive systems are designed to support one another in maintaining balance and stability.

Relative to vision, what can you, as a golfer, do to improve your core balance and stability during golf? There are two general areas I consider for a golfer, or any athlete, for that matter. There is the "hardware" side, which, simplistically, is the eyes on out, and the "software" side, or what's behind the eyes. Relative to the "hardware," the stronger and more accurate the visual signal sent by our two cameras (eyes), the better the "software" side will be able to function, resulting in more timely and accurate response, including balance.

Our research on thousands of athletes from virtually every sport and level of play indicates that athletes generally see differently than nonathletes, that higher-level athletes see differently than lesser-level athletes, and that it can even vary by position. We know that golfers are among the most visually sensitive athletes. The best LPGA and PGA golfers we've evaluated tend to "see" things that most other athletes don't. Over the years I've evaluated professional golfers that see detail far beyond the best of the best in other sports. Those golfers frequently state that one of their greatest assets is that they "see" details on the green that their peers don't. Our research also shows that virtually all visuals skills, including visually guided balance, peak in the teenage years, and begin a gradual descent in the twenties and early thirties, with a rapid drop-off in the late thirties and forties. For those golfers who are older than forty-five, you know that feeling when your arms are no longer long enough to read the scorecard at the 19th hole! These age-related visual changes can be influenced by intervention on the "hardware" and/or "software" side.

Receiving the Appropriate Vision Evaluation

For visually guided balance to be most stable, the total visual system must be operating at peak efficiency. First and foremost the "hardware" must be evaluated and any limitations corrected. Without such intervention the "software" skills, including balance, can never be fully operational.

Relative to the visual "hardware" I first recommend that the golfer receives a comprehensive vision exam, not eye exam, by a knowledgeable vision care practitioner (VCP) who "sets the vision performance bar" higher, and evaluates far more than just acuity (clarity of sight: 20/20 or 6/6, and so on); presence of nearsightedness, farsightedness, or astigmatism; and eye health. The VCP should also evaluate, at *minimum,* such skills as two-eye use, depth perception at a distance, and eye-movement and fixation skills. Visual acuity should be maximized and balanced between the two eyes for maximal depth perception, spatial awareness, and balance. Most eye care practitioners do not apply a different standard to golfers or other athletes versus the average patient. But the visual and environmental demands are far greater and unique for athletes than nonathletes.

There Is a Solution

If a vision correction is deemed appropriate I attempt to place every golfer, no matter what age, into single vision soft contact lenses, preferably a daily disposable option. Daily disposable contact lenses provide maximal comfort and clarity for every round. Contact lenses are superior to traditional spectacle corrections from both environmental and optical standpoints. There are no problems with lens reflections, fogging, sweat, foreign debris, surface scratches, frame or lens weight, frame interference, pressure points, or optical distortions with contact lenses. Blurry vision, optical distortions inherent with prescription lenses, and frame interference can have detrimental effects on golf performance, including stability and balance.

Vision/Balance Relationship Exercise #2

Peripheral vision is critical to balance/stability. With your hands in the form of fists, create small tunnels to view through. While standing on one foot fixate on a distant target straight ahead at eye level. While maintaining fixation on the distant target and continuing to stand on one foot, slowly bring both fists up directly in front of your eyes blocking all peripheral vision, similar to a pair of binoculars. You will note that balance/stability becomes stressed.

The Impact of Bifocals on Golf Performance

For those about fifty years old and now wearing some form of eyewear with a bifocal (or "no line") prescription for daily use, such a near vision correction is unnecessary, and possibly performance limiting, in golf. The bifocal generally blurs sight beyond the reading distance, therefore blurring the ball and clubhead. To avoid the blur, the golfer then makes a compensatory change in head orientation to see clearly around the blur zone, resulting in a changed posture, balance, and swing mechanics. Such a prescription distorts the periphery resulting in false spatial information, which can lead to instability and balance issues. Our research has shown that the visual demands of golf do not require a near prescription during play to see clearly. Normally, the only near demand during a round of golf is the scorecard. In the bright outdoors our pupils are smaller than indoors, resulting in greater depth of focus (or field) and the ability to see clearer much closer to oneself, including the scorecard.

Golf, reliant upon visual precision in many angles of gaze, is an endurance sport in that it is played for hours under extremes in environmental conditions, including glare and shadow. Many golfers who wear sunglasses park their eyewear on the top of their caps, particularly on the green, because the optics, tint, or frame interferes or distorts their vision. A golf-specific pair of sun eyewear is recommended to filter out potentially harmful radiation from the sun, such as UV and blue light, to allow the golfer to be more comfortable, and to provide better clarity of the golfing environment. As discussed previously, prescription eyewear has inherent optical distortions that can effect judgment of critical visual information on the course. But, even nonprescription eyewear includes varying levels of distortion, which can result in inaccurate reads of the green. Nike's golf-specific eyewear incorporates technologies to address the limitations of optics, tint, and frame interference and comfort. (Go to www.NikeVision.com for specific product solutions.)

Types of Lenses

The lens tint must allow one to see safely, comfortably, and accurately. For those of you who currently wear or have considered wearing polarized sun eyewear, this technology can limit golf performance. First, it slightly reduces visual clarity due to its composition. Second, it reduces the amount of critical visual information coming off of each blade of grass, which varies with angle of gaze, head orientation, angle relative to the changing angles/directions of the sun, and contour of the green. Polarized lenses were developed for the fishing industry. They reduce the harsh glare off the water, but unfortunately, when on land, they induce variability, an enemy of the golfer.

What about the darkness or lightness of the tint? While snow reflects approximately 85 percent of light, and cement approximately 45 percent, grass reflects only 3 to 7 percent. Therefore, to best capture the critical information reflecting off each blade of grass for contour recognition, a golf-specific lens tint should be much lighter in shade than general-use sunglasses. General-use lens tints, which are fairly dark in appearance, transmit only about 13 to 15 percent of the light reaching the eyewear. A golf-specific tint should reflect more than 20 percent, in the range of 23 to 25 percent. In summary, a golf-specific nonpolarized tint that transmits only the critical colors of the blades of grass, ball, and other surrounds, and is lighter in density than traditional tints, is recommended.

Vision/Balance Relationship Exercise #3

Think of polarized lenses as a type of venetian blind to filter out reflected glare. While wearing polarized sunglasses, standing near water facing the sun with bright glare reflected, tilt your head back and forth toward each shoulder as if to pour water out of your ear. You will notice the harsh glare alternating between an uncomfortably bright and a more comfortably dim reflection. Next, repeat the demo while standing near the edge of a green with varying contours, and facing toward the sun at a relative low angle. You will notice variability of the appearance of the grass and perceived topography.

Lastly, the position of the head and angle of gaze can influence depth perception and balance. Looking straight ahead is dramatically different than looking to the right or left while holding the head in a downward direction and lateral position while putting. Exercising these various physical and ocular postures for improved efficiency is recommended.

Vision/Balance Relationship Exercise #4

While standing on one foot (alternating right or left) tilt head from a straight-ahead gaze to the putting posture and feel the pulling sensation and decreased stability. Gradually exaggerate the angles of head torsion and angles of visual gaze. Hold the gaze. You will feel an even greater pulling sensation and instability.

ANATOMY OF THE FEET AND FOOT FUNCTION

There are nineteen muscles, thirty-three joints, and one hundred ligaments responsible for flexion, extension, and rotation of the feet and ankles. In a typical round of golf you will walk four to five miles, climb in and out of bunkers, and maneuver through difficult lies.

When a new client comes to my studio I perform a comprehensive series of assessments. The first step is to evaluate their posture, and that always begins with a diagnosis of their feet. Dysfunction in the feet directly affects knee, hip, and lumbar spine mobility and stability. As we begin our setup, the first movement is to set our stance by aligning the feet. 3D analysis proves the golf swing begins from the ground up and travels to the lower body, hips, torso, shoulders, and hands. Any dysfunction in the feet inhibits the efficiency of the kinematic sequence and transference of force.

In addition to the obvious effects of foot dysfunction on your golf game, there are many that are less obvious. For example, if you have flat feet, I can guarantee that you're also weak in your hip adductor muscle. If we focus on lifting the arches we will feel the effect directly in the adductors. The energy from the ground should travel up the legs without interruption. Flat feet cause a disruption in energy transference.

FITNESS SOLUTIONS

Note: The following exercises should be performed first with your shoes on and then with shoes removed.

Weight-Distribution-Awareness Exercise

Stand with your feet hip-width apart. Close your eyes and shift your weight forward, backward, and side to side. Return to neutral weight distribution.

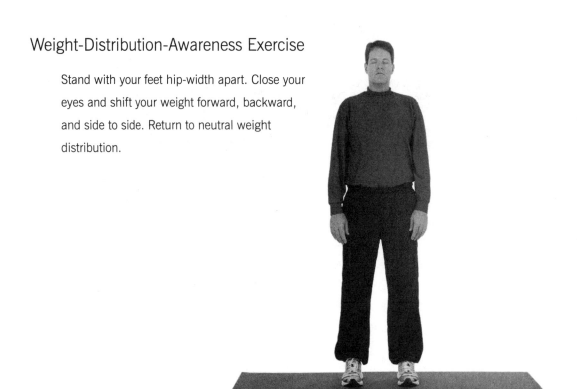

Flexion, Extension, Rotation

Flex your foot toward you, extend your foot, and rotate your foot clockwise and then counterclockwise. Repeat five times and switch sides.

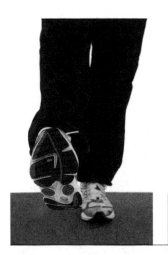 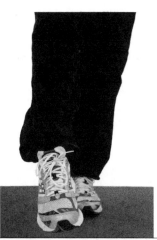

Standing Lift High Onto the Toes

Place your hands on the back of a chair. Lift yourself up
as high as you can on your toes, hold for three breaths,
and repeat five times. To make this more challenging,
place your hands by your side. To make it even harder,
close your eyes while you perform the exercise.

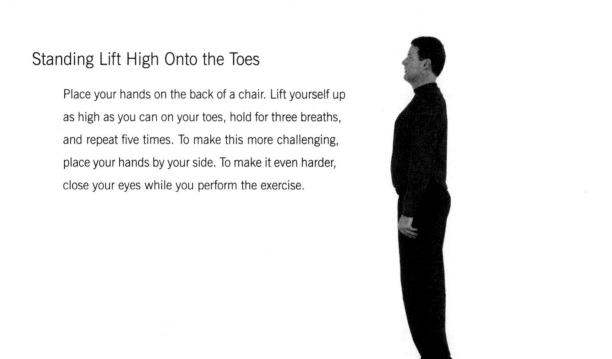

Achilles Stretch

Step back with your right foot, put your left foot forward, and place your hands on the back of a chair. Lift your right heel as high as possible, then press your right heel to the floor. Maintain the connection between your heel and the floor and bend your right knee. Focus on the stretch in the Achilles tendon at the back of your ankle. Hold for five breaths and switch sides.

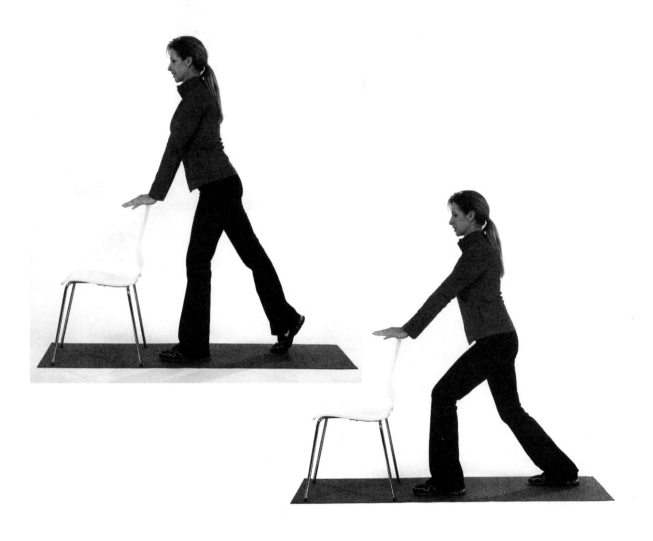

One-Leg Balance

Bring your hands to your waist and lift one leg off the floor.
Hold for thirty seconds. Switch sides and repeat the series
with the eyes closed.

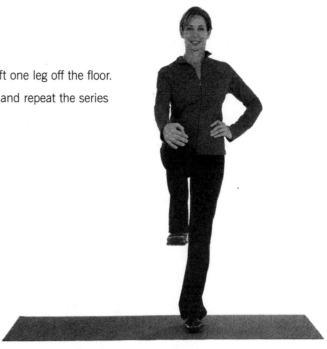

Balancing Core Series

Bring your right hand to your right knee. Hold for five breaths. Bring your right knee to the
right and hold for five more breaths. Bring your leg back to center and extend your right leg
in front of you. Hold for five more breaths. Switch sides.

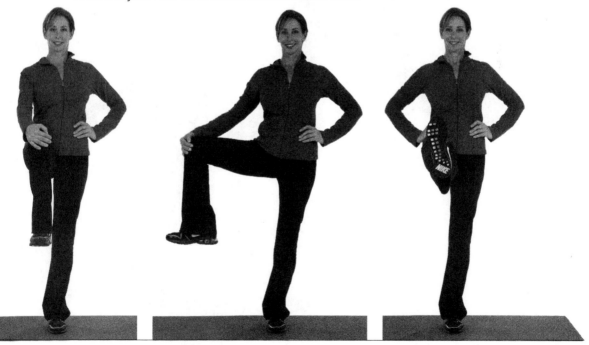

Proprioception Drill

Pay attention to the exact position and location of your left foot. Begin by shifting your weight to your right leg. Bring your right hand to the back of a chair or to the floor and lift your left leg off the floor. Hold for a few breaths and place your left foot back on the floor in the exact same position it was in when you began the exercise. Switch sides and repeat.

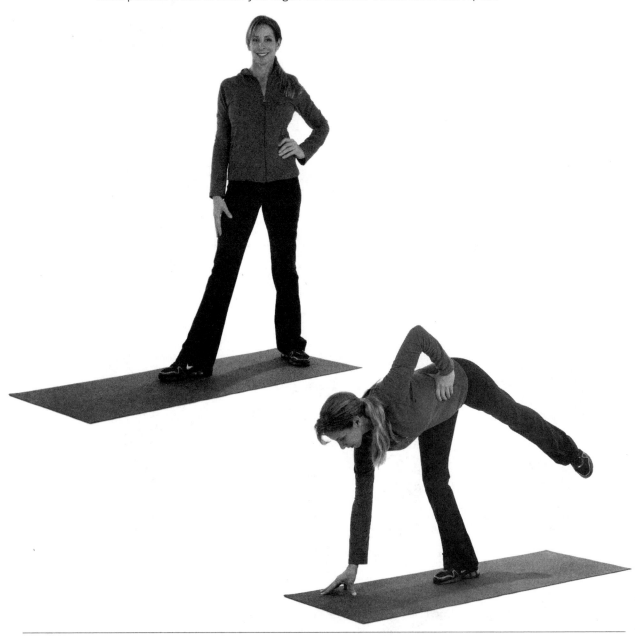

XYZ Balance Rotation Drill with Club

Extend your left leg onto a stability ball and extend your arms and club to shoulder height. Inhale, activating N.T.R., and rotate your torso over your left leg. Repeat three times and switch sides.

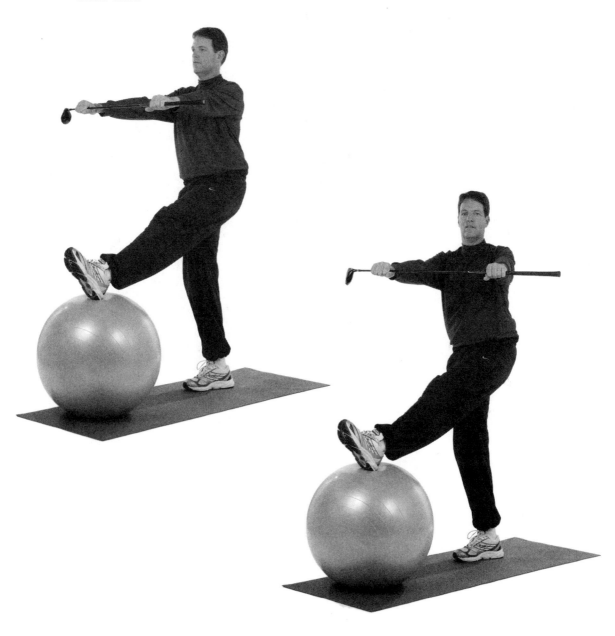

Balanced-Finish Drill

Hold your finish position for five seconds and lift your trailing leg off the floor for five more seconds.

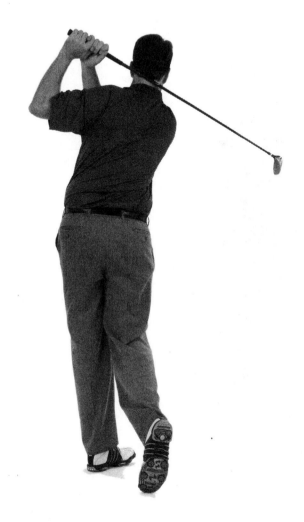

CHAPTER EIGHTEEN
THE FOUR "R"S—
RECOVER, RESTORE,
REST, AND REFUEL

I N THE PRE-ROUND warm-up chapter we specifically discussed the proper way to prepare the body for your round. We utilized "dynamic stretching," which is stretching without stopping—moving in and out of each segment of the exercise until the muscles respond. Your post-round flexibility program utilizes a different method of stretching, called passive stretching.

RECOVER

Post-round Stretching

After your round most golfers experience tension and fatigue in the muscles, primarily due to a reduction in blood flow. The by-product of this is lactic acid, which causes soreness in the muscle tissue. Post-round stretching reduces the onset of lactic acid and fatigue. Although most golfers will not take the time to stretch directly after their round (the 19th hole seems more appealing than stretching), a short series of post-round stretching exercises can reduce sore muscles and get you ready to play again.

A comprehensive post-round series targets the major muscle groups used in golf—particularly the lower back, shoulders, and hips.

A SUGGESTED LIST OF EXERCISES

Internal/External Hip Stretch

Begin with your feet wider than hip-width apart. Inhale as you bring both knees to the right.

Place your right ankle on top of your left knee. Hold for one minute and switch sides.

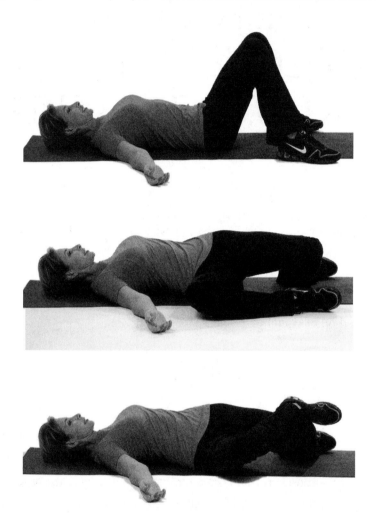

Passive and Active Elongation Hip/Quad Stretch

Place your left knee on the floor and the top of your foot against a stability ball. Slide your right knee forward until your feel the stretch in the left hip flexor and quad. Hold for five deep

breaths. To make this more challenging, you can move to the maximum range of motion in the stretch and press your foot into the ball. Hold for five breaths. Switch sides.

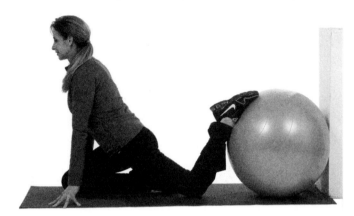

Lat Stretch

Begin by sitting on your heels, with your knees on the ground. (If you have discomfort in your knees, place a rolled up towel behind them.) Stretch your arms forward, shoulder-width apart, until they touch the floor in front of you, then go up onto your fingertips. Stretch your arms to the right, bringing your right arm perpendicular to your right hip. Maintain the connection between your left glute and your left heel. Hold for five breaths and switch sides.

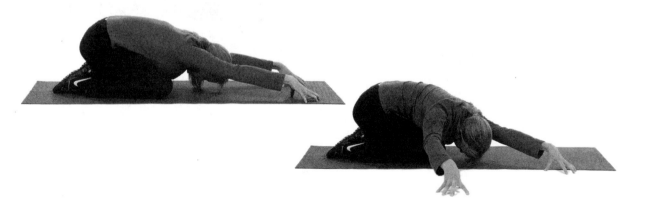

Supine Chest Stretch on the Ball

Roll a stability ball behind your upper spine, supporting your head. Lift your hips and engage your glutes until your lower body is parallel to the floor. Your arms should be at a 90-degree angle, pressing away from the ceiling, and you should be focusing on the stretch in the pecs.

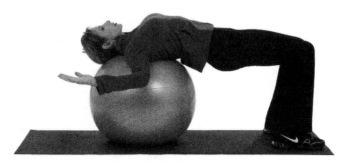

Supine Shoulder Mobility/Lumbar Stretch

Lie on your back and place your right foot on your left knee and your left hand on your right knee, then rotate your body to the left and bring your right arm to shoulder height. Hold for five deep breaths and switch sides. To make this more challenging, reach your arm over your head.

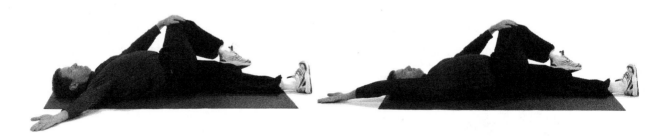

Supported Groin Stretch

Sit with your back against a wall and the soles of your feet together. Bring your feet as close as possible to your groin and hold for three minutes.

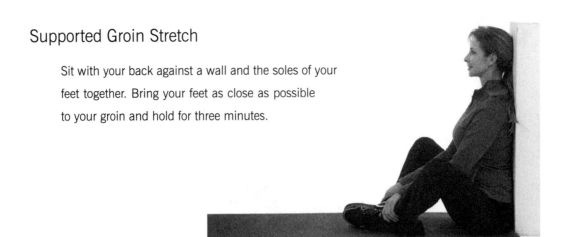

RESTORE AND REST

Rest is not appreciated in our society. Humans are the only mammals who do not nap on a regular, daily basis. Many of us push so hard to be better, play better, make more money, and run the kids around to every after-school activity that when we finally get to bed we are mentally and physically exhausted.

Rest provides an opportunity for introspection and allows us to develop clarity around our goals. As far as golf performance and fitness are concerned, we become stronger when we allow for periods of rest between our workouts and practice time. When the body is at rest, we are in a state of rejuvenation and healing. If we go to bed with shortened and tight muscles, we are aiding muscular imbalances. When we lengthen the muscles before bed, we have the opportunity to heal the muscles at the optimal length.

Here is a pre-rest series of "restorative" stretches. I use this series of exercises on a daily basis for muscular release as well as to place my body and mind in a state of rest and rejuvenation. If you experience high levels of stress, I strongly recommend using one or two of these stretches before bedtime, even if you did not play golf that day. These stretches are especially useful for traveling golfers. Use this series two hours before bedtime. But don't use muscle activation while practicing these exercises. Use your deep breathing and the force of gravity to move you deeper into the stretch. Visualize the muscles releasing with each exhalation. Close the eyes. Hold each exercise for three to five minutes.

Passive Spinal Rotation

Begin by lying on your back with your arms perpendicular to your body. Bend your knees and cross your left leg over your right. Bring your legs to the right while you maintain contact between the floor and your left shoulder. Place a towel under your knees if your knees aren't touching the floor. Rest in this position for three minutes and switch sides.

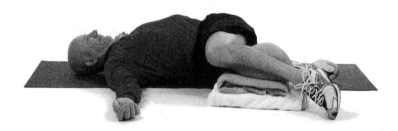

Legs up the Wall

Bring your left glute against the wall. Shift your body so your legs are on the wall, with your entire spine and hips on the floor. If your neck bothers you, place a towel under your head. To stretch your groin, bring the soles of your feet together.

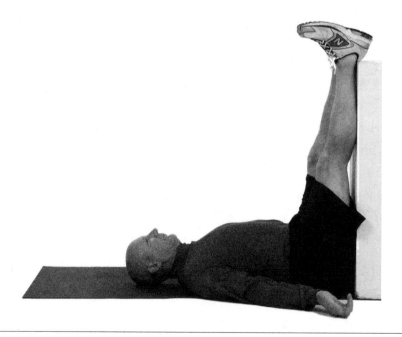

Supine Groin Stretch

Begin on your back, then bring the soles of your feet together with your palms facing the ceiling. Place towels under your knees.

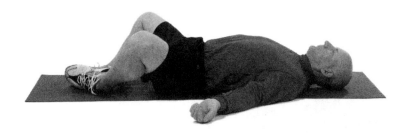

Passive Hip Release with One Leg on the Chair

Place your left leg on the seat of a chair and extend your right leg to the floor. Hold for three to five minutes and switch sides.

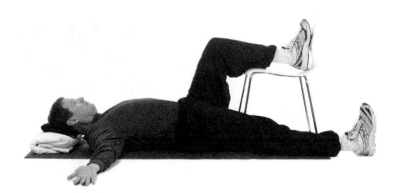

Passive Supine Chest Expansion

Lie down with a rolled-up towel under your entire spine, from the base to your head. Your knees should be bent and your palms facing up. Relax in this position while you practice ten to twenty diaphragmatic breaths. As a variation, you can extend your legs, placing the rolled-up towel under your knees.

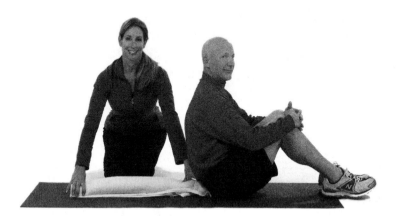

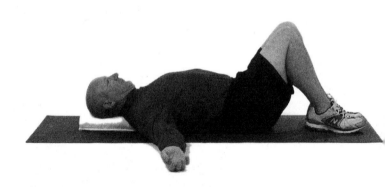

REFUEL

Proper nutrition and hydration are crucial for peak performance. Tour players often grab a snack and drink water during the round. Research has proven that nutrition affects the chemistry and function of the brain, as well as the muscle systems—proper nutrition helps you maintain flexibility, and it also reduces muscle fatigue and soreness after the round.

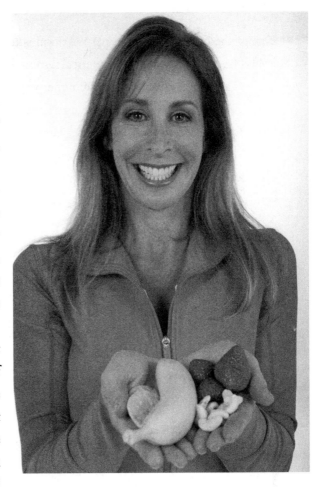

When you consider that the average round of golf is between four and five hours long (which doesn't include travel time to the course and time spent on the practice tee) you need to prepare nutritionally. You probably prepare for your round now by filling your golf bag with Band-Aids, analgesics, golf balls, and the appropriate apparel. Why not also prepare by bringing along the fuel necessary to sustain your physical and mental energy?

The Glycemic Index

One of the many goals of proper nutrition is to maintain a consistent blood-sugar level. The glycemic index is a numerical system that measures how fast a carbohydrate triggers a rise in blood sugar—the higher the number, the greater the blood-sugar spike. A low-glycemic-index food causes a small rise in blood sugar; a high-glycemic-index food causes dramatic rises (and, later on, crashes) in blood sugar.

Here are some suggestions for proper nutrition and hydration before and during your round:

Consume low-glycemic foods like oatmeal and other foods devoid of white flour or sugar. Complex carbohydrates sustain you longer than simple sugars.

Consume proteins such as chicken breasts and turkey.

Carry raw nuts (almonds and cashews) in your golf bag.

Avoid foods such as bagels, white potatoes, corn chips, pretzels, and sugary muffins (cake in disguise).

Hydration

Remaining hydrated is essential for physical and mental performance. Dehydration can cause muscular and mental fatigue, dizziness, and disorientation. Often we are not aware of dehydration until it is too late. Remember that hydration is equally as important in cold weather climates as well as warm weather conditions. Hydrate *before* you feel thirsty. Avoid dehydrating beverages such as caffeine and alcohol. Ingest eight ounces of water or electrolyte-replacement products (select a product low in sugar content) every three to four holes.

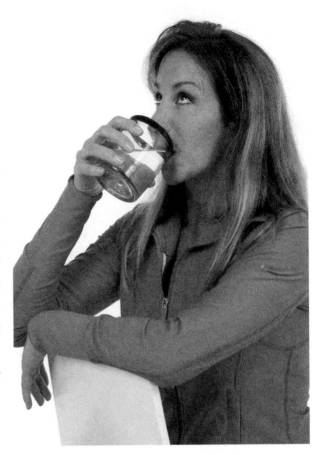